Strange I

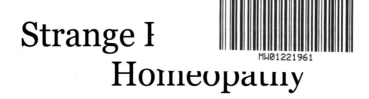

MW01221961

Homeopathy

By
Isuret Polos

First Edition

Copyright by Isuret Polos 2018

ISBN-13: 978-1986999373

ISBN-10: 1986999378

Dedicated to my father

Content

Foreword

I learned not to talk about the strange phenomenons I experience every day. At least not with everyone.

Before I talk with someone about the deeper aspects of homeopathy, I try to understand if they really want to know. Even if they are experienced homeopaths, they need to show a certain understanding for the different worldviews (*paradigms*), before I mention some of the strange phenomenons and my insights deriving from observation and study.

Writing this book is a relieve for me. You can imagine how hard it is to find someone to whom you can talk freely about the strange events I experience every day. Therefore, I will not hold myself back, or restrain myself while writing my thoughts down in an unleashed stream of words. Else I would explode and this would end in a huge mess.

Dear reader, you may be aware that homeopathy appears strange if your scientific worldview is not able to describe the true nature of consciousness.

Let me introduce you into a really strange world, if you are willed to learn, and let me show what homeopathy alone is able to provoke and shake at the base of your own worldview. If it feels strange to you, then your worldview needs probably an upgrade. On the other side only, few people accept such phenomenons like *synchronicity* or *nonlocality* as normal in the western culture, but there is indeed a wind of change blowing. In contrast to 20 years ago many people now are acquainted with concepts like *morphic resonance*, synchronicity or quantum entanglement. Materialistic science is losing territory day by day and so many people are just sick of the arrogance of an establishment which denies the existence of the free will, an elementary aspect of human being which everyone experiences on daily basis and cannot be denied! New paradigms are at the doorstep and waiting patiently to replace the old ones.

The goal of this book is to give an overview of strange phenomenons experienced by homeopathic practitioners and their patients and possible scientific explanations. It will analyse the role of a worldview based on *consciousness as the root of physical reality* and how it makes more sense to adapt to this worldview.

In the end the strange will become normal.

This book is not an introduction to homeopathy and even if it contains information about health and illnesses, therapies and remedies, it is not a substitution for a trained doctor. Your health is your own personal responsibility! I will not take any responsibility! And if you suffer from severe mental illness it would be best to stop immediately reading this book, this includes also the inclination to be overly materialistic, dogmatic or pseudoskeptic about everything or first and foremost if you suffer from religious mania (the other extreme)!

CHAPTER ONE

Strange enough

There's nothing in it

Or simply said:
"6.0221409×10^{23}"

Succussion is the process of *potentization*, by vigorously shaking with impact the properly diluted homeopathic remedy. Hahnemann believed that *succussion* and *trituration* was more important than mere dilution. The origin of succussion as a process is a bit obscure. Where did Hahnemann get the idea to add additional *kinetic energy* to the dilution process?

> The process of vigorous-shaking was known to Hahnemann before he systemized homoeopathy. But why did he use the term succussion instead of simply calling it shaking? History reveals that the term 'succussion' was used in the era of Hippocrates (460 BC – 377 BC), the Greek Physician regarded as Father of Medicine. Succussion was described by Hippocrates as a technique that consisted of shaking a patient to detect any fluid in the cavities of the body, particularly the lungs. Hippocrates insisted that the succussion process must be a firm and sudden shake; each shake should be equal in the extent of force, and those who perform it must be well trained. So how did Hippocrates came up with his technique of succussion? The answer is in his careful observation of the mechanism of cough! It is known that cough and its succussive mechanism has a forceful speed up to 50 miles per hour (about 80 Km/h). Thus Dr. Hahnemann used the term succussion to convey the essence of vigorous force that is needed in shaking the liquid to create the friction and kinetic energy that is needed for potentization.
> (Iman Navab, Reflection on trituration and succussion, *President of the Applied Research in Homeopathy Foundation of Canada*)

Typical for the materialistic science is the believe that everything is made of atoms. Newtonian science is called *atomism*, because they believe that everything can be explained by the interaction of particles. If a certain phenomenon is not explainable with atoms, well then, they expect that smaller particles may be responsible for the effect. Scientists who are stuck on this level of restricted worldview invest incredible amounts of energy, time and money to investigate smaller and smaller particles. They even assumed that a kind of "*god particle*" must exist. Imagine their frustration.

Among competing hypotheses, the one with the fewest assumptions should be selected or when you have two competing theories that make exactly the same predictions, the simpler one is the better. This is known as *Occam's razor*, a problem-solving principle attributed to William of Ockham.

Following this principle, we can analyse the simplicity of some hypothesis. Atomism is *too complicated* and therefore we can exclude this theory from the collection. Let me explain. If people invest billions of dollars for *particle accelerators*, this hypothesis cannot be the best explanation. At the most they provide cool background stories for science fiction movies.

In this case the simpler explanation is that physical reality is generated by an *immaterial* and nonlocal spirit or mind. Idealism assert that *reality is fundamentally mental*, mentally constructed, or otherwise immaterial.

What do we know from experiments, especially from *quantum mechanics*? Reality is at a certain point *fuzzy* and does not behave at all as a particle system. Instead it switches over to *probability waves*. This wave collapses to particles if they are "*observed*" or measured. This makes no sense for a Newtonian scientist. They even tried to get rid of *quantum entanglement* and nonlocality, claiming that there must be some *hidden variables* somewhere, some kind of unknown particle.

> As a man who has devoted his whole life to the most clearheaded science, to the study of matter, I can tell you as a result of my research about the atoms this much: There is no matter as such! All matter originates and exists only by virtue of a force which brings the particles of an atom to vibration and holds this most minute solar system of the atom together. . . . We must assume behind this force the existence of a *conscious and intelligent Spirit*. This Spirit is the matrix of all matter.
> (Max Planck, The Nature of Matter, 1944)

Now let's go back to the succussion or trituration process in homeopathy, which is fundamental for the production of homeopathic remedies.

What is the difference between succussion and dilution?

If you dilute a substance with water it just gets weaker. For example, if you take a poison like *Aconitum*, only 20ml of the tincture will lead to death within two to six hours. In Slovenia the folk medicine uses a daily dosage of 3 µg. One microgram is one millionth of a gram (1×10⁻⁶). A corresponding homeopathic potency would be the C3 or the D6, which is analogue to a dilution of 1:1.000.000.

But the strange phenomenon observed for the first time by Hahnemann himself was that the remedy becomes stronger with *higher potencies*.

Now a potency is *not a simple dilution*, but a dilution with additional succussion or trituration. *Kinetic force is applied.*

Aconitum is used by homeopaths usually in a higher potency like a C200 or C1000. The observed effect is, that it's curative action last longer, acts faster and it reaches deeper "*layers*".

> "But with time there emerges ever more clearly the view that, by shaking and trituration, a uniform mixing, dilution and weakening of the medicinal substance is not all that is achieved; on the contrary, the material part of the medicine is thereby more and more eradicated and as a consequence the *spiritual part* of the medicine (not perceptible to human faculties) is released and *extraordinarily* increased. This is *dynamization* ... be possible to increase the power by succussion; the more the medicine is succussed when prepared, the stronger its effect ..." [Haehl, 1922, vol.1, p.324]

How could this be possible in a world where particles bounce against each other and make things somehow happen? Materialism is a *contradictory science* which applies *reductionism* in an exaggerated manner, isolating everything from its context and by doing this they exclude the meaning of all they try to explore.

Occam's razor would require a *simpler explanation*. Try to put consciousness in the centre of the universe, just for fun. If the physical universe is based on pure consciousness, then I promise you, it will make all more sense. Not only regarding homeopathy, but also all the other crazy stuff like quantum entanglement, teleportation, nonlocality, levitation, and who knows what other things. Maybe you have personally experienced stuff like *telepathy*, *clairvoyance*, *psychokinesis* and so on. How could this possible fit into a materialistic world?

As a homework, put the materialistic worldview away for some months and try to view through the "*idealism glasses*". It's your freedom of choice to switch a worldview or point of view temporarily. It should not hurt you in anyway. Just try it out!

Homeopathic remedies are still entangled to the original substance. If the original substance does not exist anymore, like a radioactive substance which is already decayed, transmuted into a lighter element, then how would this entanglement be possible?

Again, Occam's razor, idealism, not materialism. The idea of the original substance still exists in an immaterial realm. Why should pure consciousness forget something? It does not depend on material brains or hard-disks or laser-discs. *It is nonlocal*!

Rupert Sheldrake explains his own observations with his *morphic resonance theory*. Invisible and immaterial morphic fields are responsible for the *formative process* in embryos, how single cells forms a complex organ, even how substances generate *crystals*. This morphic fields exists independently of the material counterpart. Sheldrake's theory is very similar to idealism. And it explains a lot more than a materialistic attempt.

But how is it possible that the morphic field of say Aconitum entangles with the water or sugar during succussion or trituration? Because you need to know that there are remedies like Aqua, which is pure water, or Saccharum, potentized sugar. How is it possible that during succussion of Aconitum the morphic field of this toxic plant is bound to the water without the morphic field of the water itself? And how can you isolate the morphic field of sugar during a trituration?

Again, Occam's razor, the simplest answer is: *Intention*!

Because physical reality is based on consciousness, the intention of the laboratory assistant is the key factor. They potentize the original substance and during the first potencies they *bind* it's morphic field to the *carrier material*. They may be aware of it or not. But fact is, the first few hours of trituration and succussion are crucial and can be regarded as a *ritual of binding*.

This works so well, that in the so called *"C4 Homeopathy"* only trituration is applied, even to liquid substances. Usually practitioners of homeopathy meet at a trituration "party" where they triturate a known or unknown remedy for the first time. During this process they experience *the essence of the remedy* themselves. At the beginning the C1 provokes physical symptoms. The next day or next week they triturate the C2 and usually they have emotional symptoms. When they triturate the C3 mind symptoms appears. And these movement has the goal to go further, to reach at least the C4, which means that one experience symptoms on the so called *"spiritual level"*, where the core essence of the remedy is expressed.

Consciousness is essential
Binding of a morphic field to the milk sugar is not done on a physical level. There are methods which proves this. A little warning, do not search for proof inside the *materialistic science framework*, because this would prove just one thing: that you have not understood the difference between these two worldviews! Materialism is not able at all to explain the spirit or the true nature of consciousness. It is limited to the physical realm.

The question arises if it is possible to use intention only, get rid of the physical and go straight to the core of a remedy?

The simple answer is yes, it is possible. But who has this ability to use it intentionally? There may be a time in life when one admires nature and has this *blissful moments* and a *healing process* is initiated. During this moment you feel the *energy flow* in your *meridians, goose bumps, electricity,* and certain *insights* or *visions* may arise. It's like the sun shines inside you.

But to use pure intention only is a *rare art*. The problem is, that we are all ill. How can a blind man help another blind man? Certain religious sects and organisations practice *"faith healing"* exploiting credulous people. Where money flows abundantly, there is no free flow of life force, because money replace spirit with *greed*.

Anyway, intention is required in many healing arts. For example, without intention acupuncture does not work properly. There is always the need of a *framework* and knowledge of human anatomy, psychology and its *energetic system*. In *acupuncture* a needle can sedate or tonify a meridian if inserted in one and the same point. The difference between sedation or tonification is achieved by the "*manipulation of the needle*". Here plays the intention a major role than the selection of the acupuncture point.

CHAPTER TWO

Higher Order

From above downwards.
From within outwards.
From a more important organ
to a less important one.
In the reverse order of their coming.

What renders physical reality stable if it is just a *mental construct*?

We regard an idea as very volatile as long it is not written down on a piece of paper or even carved in stone. Remember the ten commandments? The second time Moses went down from the mountain his face was emitting rays. Because of their importance the ten commandments were written in stone, not because they were volatile in their true nature. Jesus said that the ten commandments (including the whole Law and the Prophets) are based on just two commandments or principles, to love God and to love your neighbor as yourself.

Principles are eternal. They do not decay and they do not become less important with time. Indeed, *a spirit is stronger than a physical body*. It's an illusion that physical reality is more stable than mental constructs. Only materialists believe in a supremacy of matter. It would be fool to believe that 2 comes before 1. So, spirit, the immaterial and the nonlocal, is prior to matter.

A materialist denies the father, because the mother (from Latin "*mater*", meaning mother) is more important for them. Here lies the core of modern human society after the fall. Cush, known by other folks as the god of chaos, was the father of Nimrod. Because Cush was a Baal worshipper, a proponent of the first state demonic religion of Babel, he was expected to sacrifice his firstborn male child. Doing this they would prevent that the messiah would ever born and doing this they would perpetuate human rulership. *Semiramis* the wife of Cush, known also as *Ishtar*, knew that she needed to hide their firstborn. Therefore, she gave his son to another family far away. When Nimrod grew up he returned to Babel just in time to witness a confusion of divine origin. People started to talk in different languages. And this confusion leads also to rivalry between the clans and to fighting about resources and territory. During this confusion Nimrod killed his own father Cush. Later he married Semiramis, unaware that she was his own mother. Semiramis and Nimrod ruled together over the remaining clans. Nimrod trained the first soldiers for the purpose of war, the *very first wars* ever fought. So, he became a kind of prototype for a leader in this materialistic world. He destroyed during his war campaigns and his mother rebuild the society according to her will. She was the mother goddess, the goddess of heaven, worshipped and adored. Today we

14

observe this misbehaviour when a country attacks another country, claiming to help them. War and crime is the promoter of materialism. A system where money is the blood, war is the heart. There will be never peace in a world based on materialism. And science cannot achieve new insights if their axiom is still based on materialism, denying the father, denying spirit, the invisible and nonlocal.

Now enough of the history lesson. Back to the strange phenomenons we can observe in homeopathy.

What we can observe is a certain direction of healing. This phenomenon is not limited to homeopathy, but every true healing art is able to observe it. It denotes a hidden law.

From above downwards
The free will and the dignity of a human being is more important than his toes. In some way the *life force* arranges and *orders chaos*, limiting it to less important parts of human anatomy. The brain is more important than the skin. His heart is more important than the muscular system. From above downwards is the *direction of healing*. Observed by Hahnemann himself for the first time, written down as part of set of a "*rule*" or "*law*" by Constantine Hering, or at least attributed to him as the "author" of the so-called law, this is a very strange phenomenon from a materialistic point of view. But think about it, how is the human anatomy designed? Bones acts as shields, especially for the brain and lungs and heart. So why should an invisible force act contrary? It's natural that the energetic system protects the body from worse illness by limiting the damage to the periphery.

Many practitioners observed a shift of the symptoms from the head, or even from the mind, towards the extremities, when the right remedy was prescribed. And finally, when the cure was complete, it reached the skin and then dissolved there to a state of wellbeing.

Here you can observe that the *intention* of the life force is to protect the spirit in first place, the organs which host the spirit and interacts with it, to protect the *free will* and the *dignity* or *heart* (centre of the being). Lesser parts can be sacrificed if necessary. There is an intelligence embedded in our life force.

This phenomenon delivers a hint for why physical reality seems so stable. The spirit knows something, a master plan, an *interwoven network of energetic rivers*, with nodes linked to each other. Consciousness is at the base of it. And because the base is eternal, the *awareness for eternity* exists in us. The life force is able to repair damage to this network, as long as there is no *obstruction* to the *free flow*.

An illusion is a blockage to the truth and the free flow of life force.

For example, a typical case of *Ignatia*. They may believe they have lost someone or something for good and they will never be united again. The feeling of a lump in their throat, an energetic blockage of the *throat chakra*, dissolves during the healing process, removing the obstacle for free speech. Later the blockage in the stomach dissolves, removing the obstacle to assimilate food. Expressing their feelings is regarded more important than the assimilation of food. Therefore, the order from throat to stomach. Ignatia is known for many kinds of eating disorders, but it is also known for their emotional sensitivity and their *silent grief*.

From the very beginning of homeopathy, symptoms in the materia medica and in most repertories are listed from mind to head to the feed, always from above downwards. I don't know not even one exception to this rule. It's an intrinsic attribute of homeopathy.

From within outwards
Very similar to the first aspect of the law, from above downwards, the *"from within outwards"* is the direction which a cure takes also. And this is interesting, because it is to 100% conform with the first aspect of the law. It renders a *3-dimensional picture* of the *dynamic* of a healing process. We have the x,y and z vectors, but there is more. Both two aspects are embedded inside the third, *"from a more important organ to a less important one"*.

In the reverse order of their coming
This is the only aspect which seems not to fulfil always. Because an old symptom does not need to reappear if the healing process is fast enough. Whole stages can be skipped, especially during acute illness. Generally said, the last aspect of Hering's law is more a practical rule, because not every symptom is really reversible, but it is for sure a good sign if the healing takes this direction.

Even if many homeopaths regard Hering's law as a "*normal pattern*", I find the last aspect raver intriguing. It denotes some kind of memory for the chronicle of the illness. As if the body remembers the order of the appearing of symptoms and it is able to play them back to the beginning.

Another explanation is, that the order is simple bound to aspect one and two of the law, say to "*from above downwards*" and "*from within outwards*".

CHAPTER THREE

Dreams

Heh, heh ... what's happened to me?
I must be dreaming.
I feel like I can take out the world.
(Tetsuo)

There is nothing more real than reality, except *lucid dreams*.

The proving of *Phosphorus* C1000 revealed as the most potent *lucid dream* stimulator. A few globulis and the clarity of my dreams enhanced in such a way, that I became *aware that I was dreaming*. Everything felt so real. The wind, the cold dark water, the stars, the dirt on the ground, the food, the flesh and the fire. It was impossible to tell if it was true or not, because it was more real than reality.

Under the influence of the energy of Phosphorus the borders between you and me, between this world and the immaterial world, between wake and dream are blurred. Sympathy is overly exaggerated and becomes the ability to get in resonance with everything. The nervous system becomes a high frequency antenna and it receives broadcasting signals from everywhere. Vivid dreams, lucid dreams, persistent dreams. Phosphorus is the dream remedy number one!

In one dream, still under the influence of Phosphorus, I dreamed of giant ants. They were all over my bed, huge like dogs, and when one of them bite me it was so painful, you cannot imagine. On waking up the pain lasted few seconds and then vanished. The materia medica says *"dreams of stinging insects"*.

Our brain consists of water, fat and phosphorus. A great simplification of the three main components. Homeopathic remedies are able to stimulate our brain cells and our brain activity. During a homeopathic proving the experimenter will collect as many symptoms as possible, which includes mind symptoms, impressions and dreams. Especially dreams are interesting, because they are connected to the collective unconsciousness.

It may happen, that a dream becomes true. One night I got this dream: I stood on a river in middle of a forest, the water flowed backward. An old man was near a bed. In the bed was a woman holding a baby. In the background I saw a floor clock which went also backward. When I woke up from the dream I was in a sad mood. Later on, the same day a friend gave me a DVD and told me that this movie is crazy and I should watch it. So, it revealed that my dream was about the movie *"The Curious Case of Benjamin Button"*, a man who starts aging backwards, born as an old man and becoming younger with time, ending his life as a baby. The next day

I asked my friend a few questions. When did he decide to give me the DVD? Was he thinking about me when he watched the movie? It was no coincidence. He really decided to give me the movie, because he was curious how I would react to it. This can be regarded as telepathy or more specific a kind of dream telepathy. A sender and a receiver. I believe that this kind of telepathy only worked because my friend was firm in his decision to give me the movie on the next day and that I would watch it. This kind of interconnection requires a potential in order to create the transmission of this information. The potential was a combination of his decision and my acceptance to watch the movie. Else I would have just dreamed of pink ponies as usual.

I experimented with Phosphorus quit a lot, but I needed to stop eventually, because besides of stomach pain it makes you sensitive to every atmospheric change. At a certain point one gets over sensitive to a remedy.

Thinking of dream telepathy, could it be used to send any kind of message? There are some reports of successful experiments. But one problem is that the language during dreams belongs to the collective unconsciousness, a language based purely on *symbolism*. Abstract languages, like human language, is not available on this level of reality.

Some scientists and language experts say that symbolism is a primitive language. I regard it as a *low-level language* and not primitive. Primitive denotes that it needs to evolve in some way into a higher form, but the symbolic language is a *universal language*. It's like a programming language of a computer. There is machine code, *assembler*, a low-level programming language, and then there are *high level languages* like C++ or Python. These languages are called complex or abstract languages, but they are based on the lower level language. Our human language is a complex and abstract one too. The symbolic language is low level, but a powerful one, as machine code is a powerful language too. The machine code for example is able to address the hardware directly. In the case of symbolic language, it is able to directly address the *framework of physical reality*.

I cannot stress enough the importance of the symbolic language, because the entire materia medica revolves around symbolism and the subconscious world. I wonder if Carl Gustav Jung did know homeopathy. So, I searched in the Internet and found a wonderful article on *"Sue Young Histories"* (sueyounghistories.com), a blog which is specialized in biographies of people who was influential in homeopathy or was influenced by homeopathy. And indeed, Jung did know homeopathy:

> Jung once wrote "...regarding homeopathy, you are quite right to see it as a continuation of alchemical practice" (C. G.;Adle Jung, *Letters of C. G. Jung: Volume I, 1906-1950,* (Taylor & Francis, 17 May 1973)) and "I shall not commit the fashionable stupidity of regarding everything I cannot explain as a fraud," (C.G. Jung, *Jung on Synchronicity and the Paranormal*, (Routledge, 7 Aug 1997). Page 57.).
>
> ...
>
> Jung's concept of synchronicity tears apart cause and effect and the rationality of scientific fundamentalism, thus 'our world' is phenomenological, not empirical.
>
> ...
>
> Jung believed that alchemy is a law of the psyche. Jung postulated that suggestibility, or psychic infection (or groupthink) underlies mass psychology.

Many homeopaths considered the symbolic language as a universal and powerful language. It's importance for finding the similimum is vital in difficult cases, where the communication on higher level is blocked, when abstract language is not able to express the pain and suffering anymore. Then the subconscious takes over and uses symbolism to reveal the key for healing the fractured whole.

It goes even beyond the subconscious. When the subconscious itself is blocked, it could happen that the collective subconscious intervenes. Then what is hidden inside a human being, in one individual person, is expressed by the collective, by other people in the vicinity.

I could observe this phenomenon when I took a very high potency of Lycopodium. And with high I mean a C1.000.000, or a MM, one million! Why did I take this remedy? I observed that in my family and in my surrounding (colleagues, friends, and so on) the typical theme of Lycopodium emerged. Lycopodium is the type of "*inferior*" man who loves power in order to compensate his feeling of inferiority. Most times they are really inferior in terms of physical maturity, general debilities. Their inferiority is expressed also on emotional level. Their relation to the "*father*" is weak. It makes no difference if "*father*" means the heavenly father, God or just the biological father. If their biological father was a Lycopodium type too, then he refused to take responsibility for their family and as all remedies in the tuberculosis miasm, they love to travel, travel far away from their family, far away from every responsibility. It happened that so many people resembled the Lycopodium type, that the fight for more power inside the family and in our surrounding became overwhelming. I identified more than 7 persons who was really Lycopodium types and more than 20 persons who was influenced by them. All in all, there was 120 persons who got a negative impact of this collective illness. In some way there was a centre of attraction for Lycopodium and someone was the key person for this strange phenomenon. The problem was that I could not give to anyone of them Lycopodium with the pretence to help them, because it is not right in an ethical way, even if it is "*only sugar*" from a materialistic point of view. But what I was allowed to do was to take it myself. And I did. I chose the MM potency because the problem was my surrounding. The effect was undeniable. Like an atomic explosion, me as the centre, all people around me was hit by the shock wave. They all got symptoms, on the physical, emotional, mind and spiritual level. A temporary aggravation followed by an improvement on all levels, means the Lycopodium types ... all of them, after only two months, continued their journey, to other countries or other companies, left the family and neighbourhood for good, and to be never ever seen again. The effect on me? It was easy peasy my friend. I got not even one symptom of Lycopodium. Maybe it was the right potency, only in resonance with my surrounding, or maybe because I was in the centre of this lycopodian hurricane, a region of calm weather with no wind.

The Lycopodium patient says: „*Everything I eat turns into wind*". Oh, they are so right!

What are these coincidences called, when a patient takes a remedy and symbolism of the remedy emerge in their surroundings?

We will discuss this in the next chapter.

CHAPTER FOUR

Synchronicity

"We often dream about people from whom we receive a letter by the next post. I have ascertained on several occasions that at the moment when the dream occurred the letter was already lying in the post-office of the addressee."
(C.G. Jung, Synchronicity:
An Acausal Connecting Principle)

A person takes Natrium-muriaticum, dreams of a mouse and when he wakes up there is really a mouse in his house. The mouse represents his inner state of mind, his timidity, and because the mouse is there at the same day he took the remedy, this demonstrates that an inner state was expressed by physical reality. This is what we know as synchronicity.

Synchronicity are *meaningful coincidences*. Jung describes them as *inner events* (dreams, ideas, emotions) expressed by physical events.

I experience synchronicities every day, therefore I wonder why most people don't notice them too. Sure, some people are more open to it than others, but most people are *not aware of their inner feelings*, so why should they become aware of strange correlated events too? Than more you are inclined to *observe yourself*, than more you will become aware of synchronistic events. They are similar to dreams. Everybody dreams, not everybody is able to remember them. To notice synchronicity is similar to become aware that you are in a dream. It requires almost the same amount of awareness.

For example, I took *Praseodymium* one day, because of a health issue, not for experimenting. Before I took it, I wondered if some synchronicity would occur, because I read that chemical elements from the lanthanides series has this strong magnetic force. In a forum someone wrote that he took *Neodymium*, which is also a lanthanide, and his notebook broke soon after.

Only two hours after I took Praseodymium my iMac PC broke. What a coincidence! I went to the Apple store and they told me that the graphics card which was embedded in this specific model was known to have a serious problem and it could have break anytime. I was lucky that it happened just one week before my guarantee expired.

The funny thing about all this was, that there was already a potential breakpoint. It broke only two hours I took Praseodymium and 3 hours I read that lanthanides could do this.

From a quantum mechanics point of view, this event did not break any *law of energy conservation*. The remedy just modified the time when it happened or the probability when it should happen.

When you buy a computer, should you take one dose of Praseodymium C1000 in order to make sure, that all breakpoints survive the quantum flux stress?

Joke apart, computer designer, specifically computer chips designer, has a big struggle with such occurrences. They know that *quantum tunnelling effects* can happen and therefore they try to work around with some quantum mechanics tricks or by adding more cores. Than smaller the circuit in a CPU becomes, than more *quantum leaks* occur. It's like trying to prevent electrons from *teleporting* themselves to other wires. At smaller scale quantum properties starts to emerge, because the interpretation of space location seems to lose importance and other properties like that of time gain priority.

The truth is synchronicity is not only a strange phenomenon, but it is necessary for life. Our brain would never work without synchronicity. The neurophysiologist and Nobel prize winner *Sir John Carew Eccles* was sure that a quantum entanglement between our mind and the neurons exist. He wrote in his book *"How the Self Controls Its Brain"* that neurons could fire a signal on their own during the day, without external stimulus. This could happen just once a day. The probability is very low, but it's there, somewhere higher than improbable. And then the wonder happens: we decide to raise our arm and millions of neurons fires without external stimulus from other neurons, just because our *immaterial mind* changed the *probability* when the *improbable event* occurs. While I write this book, my finger moves and hits the keys to form words and phrases, and some grammatical errors too maybe, just because events occur in a synchronistic manner, without breaking the law of energy conservation. I love when this happens. Quantum mechanics in a wet and warm environment, inside the brain, also known as quantum biology ... or coffee overdose?! ... anyway ...

20 years ago, while training in a fitness club, I took *Arnica* C200 against muscle soreness. An excellent remedy for athletes (I'm not an athlete actually, but sport is for sure real fun), besides Rhus-tox and Symphytum officinale. Jan Scholten wrote in his book

"*Wonderful Plants*" that some plants absorb elements from the earth regarding their own nature. Especially the plants from the family group Campanulidae, which contains also the *Asterales* group and as a special member Arnica montana, absorbs *lanthanides* in bigger quantities from the earth through their *roots*. This plant family has one main theme with the lanthanides in common: a strong drive for *individuality, independence* and living their own life. You can recognize this in Arnica, but also in other members of this family like Calendula, Cina and so on.

Arnica provokes synchronistic events which resembles *incidents*. When I took for the first time Arnica C200, one hour later a friend let his car keys fall down a gully. The second time I took this remedy, almost 15 years later, a policeman let also his car keys fall down. This happened after one hour I took Arnica C1000. His colleague looked at him astonished and asked him "what happens with you". You need to know that this policeman walked like Dirty Harry through the parking lot and he was for sure a typical Arnica type, strong, the "*nobody would ever touch me*" kind of man. Only 10 minutes later, I was in a store buying something to drink, a woman let her stuff fall down on the ground. The policemen were present and they both found it very amusing. It happened again, just a few weeks ago, this time with a lower potency of only C30, a woman let her stuff fall down in a store after 30 minutes I took Arnica. Well by the way, when I take Arnica, it happens to me too.

When I read my *diary*, I find more strange occurrences (always on the same day, within 24 hours):

- *Calcium phosphoricum* C10.000, one of my teeth broke while eating soup (what a loser)
- *Stramonium* C1000, a TV comedian show cancelled, but they show a horror movie instead (thank you)
- *Pulsatilla* C200, because I'm curious, and shortly after I got 3 phone calls from women living in different cities and countries, all asking what remedy they can take for the menopause

Not always I need to take the remedy. Sometimes it's more than enough to trigger synchronistic events when I study a particular remedy.

Magnesium phosphoricum is a remedy with huge problems in communication and aggression. While I was studying Jan Scholten's book "Homeopathy and Elements", I was on the chapter of Magnesium, a young boy ringed at my door. He was from Niger, talked very good German. He said he got my address from a common friend. So I invited him in, we eat some spaghetti and talked. He just wanted to spent some time with friends of his friends. I'm totally ok with that. At a certain point the conversation touched his family condition and he began to stutter. Not the occasional stutter, but a real problem was recognizable in his voice and rhythm. He could not express freely his anger towards his father. He was the victim, he said. But he was also an aggressor in some way, which he could not hide. The root cause of his problems was the recurring conflicts in his family. Whenever he talks about his family, he said, he begins to stutter. These was all Magnesium-phosphoricum themes, the stutter, aggressiveness in family, problems with communications, no stability, pain.

Not all synchronistic events are safe. Especially radioactive elements like the actinides can trigger the worst. Therefore, one cannot just play with them. Actinides are known to trigger catastrophic events, severe incidents and they do not only break electronics in the vicinity like the lanthanides, but also glass breaks.

Animal remedies attracts synchronicities which contains similitudes regarding the animal behaviour, territorial fighting or attracts the animal itself into your vicinity. When I took Tyto Alba C10.000 one day a rare coincidence occurred. I was walking home from the office. As usual I walked through the fields, because I love nature. In this fields I knew every bird, every insect and plant. And because photography is one of my hobbies too, I collected a lot of photos of different plant species. I thought I would know every living thing in this field, but when I took Tyto Alba, which is a remedy made from a feather of the barn owl, this must have attracted the rarest bird in the surroundings. On that day it has snowed, not much, but the fields were all white. And then I saw them sitting there on a tree, all three together, snowy owls, in Germany! A friend of mine is a bird expert. He told me that it's almost impossible that snowy owls would fly towards this region. Well, maybe these was not snowy owls from the arctic, but they were white owls, really beautiful. I've have never seen then again after that day when I took the remedy.

How do we make sense of synchronicity? I believe that the information of a remedy resides on the dimension of time only and there it exhibits its power, by creating order on time. Time is spaceless and therefore also immaterial. When different events happen at the same time and they have all the same theme in common, this points towards a greater meaning, a node or crossover in time where order emerge from the immaterial realm. Our consciousness as a whole generates time as a way to communicate. This must create tension between the eternal and the temporary. When the tension is too big, synchronicity occurs in order to relieve the tension and we become aware of it. In this regard synchronicity is similar to the tension between the subconscious and the consciousness, where relieve is achieved by expression of symbolic meaning during dreams.

CHAPTER FIVE

Collective Trauma

"Our ancestors dreamed us up
and then bent reality to create us."
(Walidah Imarisha)

Universal principles like that of homeopathy are key elements of the core understandings of cosmology. Whatever helps us to understand how consciousness generates physical reality as a communication platform and how it stabilizes this level, is more than precious for scientists, artists and the in between, like metaphysicians.

Every remedy, every family or group has his own theme and resonance to traumas. Some themes are a problem of just one individual person, but as many homeopaths now recognize very well, there is always a collective issue too. We are all sitting in one boat.

The collective of humanity is at a certain point one whole organism. It behaves like that, distributing resources for the greater good, cancelling out bad behaviour, building up potential for later use.

Deep inside the collective subconsciousness exists thought forms which acts like antibodies. There is an immune system embedded in the collective. We were created in a way that ensures that humanity will survive as a whole.

The normal state would be a free flow of energy inside the individual person, between persons, between the planet and other solar systems, between galaxies. And humans would live forever, with a perfect health, a sense in their life.

Something went wrong
Now there is a kind of collective amnesia. You know that kind of amnesia which only forms if a huge trauma occurred in the past.

And if this kind of trauma really exist, what would you expect happens if you address it in public? Sure, open minds would be curious, would invite you for a beer, tell us more, come on!

But the academia is stubborn, elitary and dogmatic. Try to tell them that there exists a trauma deep in our subconscious collective and that we are not anymore able to remember it.

This happened to Immanuel Velikovsky. When he used comparative mythology to prove that Earth suffered catastrophic close contact with other planets in ancient times, like Venus and Mars, the critics and hostility exploded to such an extent that some commentators have made an analysis of the conflict itself.

Some scholars refused Velikovsky's unorthodox method to use mythology for identifying cosmological events in the past. But mythology is exactly the best way to gather data from catastrophic events, because mythology is a way how consciousness handles traumatic events. If a trauma is too big, we invent a story which describes the trauma and then we pass it to the next generation. They are part of the collective too and maybe they are able to dissolve the trauma.

If life energy lacks, this means if awareness lacks or is blocked, then our consciousness refuses to elaborate a trauma. Maybe because it's dangerous to try to dissolve a trauma if one is too weak. Unfortunately, it could also happen, that when we become stronger, the trauma remains and embeds deep into the subconsciousness, becoming the new normal state.

A defence mechanism is then build around the trauma core. It's an exclusion zone, a taboo theme. If you are caught walking near the borders you will get shot immediately.

No wonders that people who tried to translate the Bible into a modern language was cut into pieces alive, mutilated, burned, hanged and not exactly in this order. Such an expression of hate can only come from someone who misuses the status quo and gains great profit from it. The Bible describes exactly what we define as the biggest traumatic event of humankind, how and why it happened, how it will be dissolved in a near future, what everyone of us need to do.

And comparative mythology is able to trace it back combining different angles.

Now what is most important in the context of this book, is the reaction of someone who is confronted with one of the many aspects of the collective trauma. Avoidance is the normal reaction. Hiding is another. And a miasmatical illness is able to camouflage itself until you hit the nail on his head. Therefore, Hahnemann was so desperate before he discovered the miasms.

Today we know a lot more miasms than Hahnemann, to be precise 18 miasms which are similar to the 18 stages of chemical elements in the periodic table. Perhaps it's no coincidence that human imperfection is described in the Bible with the number 666. But I don't want to dive into numerology right now. My supply of absinthe is unfortunately depleted.

Each miasm is a way to distribute the trauma on the collective level.

A single person has not enough power to dissolve the collective trauma. But groups of people have at least enough energy to hold the trauma stable. And in the meantime, before the trauma will be dissolved once and for all, we suffer under the influence of the miasm and we can recognize a common theme, just like mythologies has a common theme too.

For example, Niobium. It can be found in the periodic table on stage 5, series 5. Niobium is the most hounded type of creative person. It belongs to the silver series, where Argentum is the best-known remedy. They have a lot of ideas, but they are stuck in the so called "development hell". This word derives from the media industry, a jargon describing a project which remains in development for a very long time without progressing to completion. For an artist this is a painful state.

Similar to Niobium is the Malaria miasm. The common theme of Malaria is to be stuck and not able to progress and finish something. Most time they blame outer circumstances, and most time they are right, because war and conflicts are one of these circumstances which exists especially in countries where Malaria is a big issue. Most people there need remedies which relates to the Malaria miasm.

Dissolving the common theme of a miasm in a country inflicted by war and conflicts would imply a huge change on a global scale. Coward countries which hold them down deliberately with political tricks, even by mean of proxy wars, continues to gain huge profits by exploiting their mineral resources, diamantes, precious metals, oil, and so on. The entire world economy would suffer a big loss if just one of this so called "developing country" would shake away the bonds. This requires a raising of the individual awareness and that of the collective at the same time. Money would lose value because not enough people would attribute a value to it.

How reacts some countries when their power and wealth is under threat through a metaphysical medium like homeopathy? They invent new laws which restricts the practice of homeopathy. Or they start pseudoskeptics campaigns in order to defame homeopathy. It seems that only homeopathy was the target of such a coward attack. Neither acupuncture or TCM or Ayurveda or any other therapy method was so intensely attacked as homeopathy. With one exception, radionics, and quite successful.

Another example are countries where people seems to suffer under a common plant family theme. Most Italians and other Southern Europeans are in resonance with the Solanaceae, the nightshades. No wonder, because tomatoes, eggplant, bell peppers and chili peppers are all part of this family group, all essential ingredients of the Italian kitchen. Even tobacco makes part of the Solanaceae, the most consumed drug in Europe.

The Solanes main theme is the fight between the light and the dark. They fear to be a bad person. When a Mafiosi commit's his usual crime, he searches relief from his guilty conscience by confessing his sins to a priest. The Catholic Church on the other side takes advantages of their situation and transmutes the sins of the Mafiosi into money. This is the best alchemy invented by Italians.

They fear to be seen as bad. They smile, makes jokes, play the clown. Or they insist on their non-existing honour. A lot similarity to Belladonna and Hyoscyamus. Typical themes like hellfire and demons are found in the Solanaceae family members.

Witch Hunts has its roots in Europe and was exported to America. In old books the witches flying ointment is described to be a combination of 3 to 4 plants, all from the Solanaceae family, Belladonna, Hyoscyamus, Stramonium and Mandragora. A typical theme in dreams is to fly away from their problems or enemies.

Lyssinum has similarities with Stramonium. They fear the Church, church music, water (or maybe holy water?). Lyssinum should be remembered when someone suffers from religious mania.

All Solanaceae have a problem with religion, searching refuge in it without accepting the truth or gaining real knowledge. It's more a desperate primitive ritual for them, getting protection from idols like Maria, Jesus on a cross or a picture of Padre Pio. Superstition derives from a lack of true knowledge, compensating their craving for spiritual truths.

As you can see, Belladonna is not only good for treating fever or a sunburn. Homeopathy can be a lot more interesting if you combine it in an interdisciplinary way. Restricting your own knowledge by refusing to read books, claiming that you know enough, would mean that you maybe need a remedy from the Solanaceae family, because Italy and Greece ("una faccia una razza", one face one race) are known for not reading books, remaining in the dark, under the shadow of the night, bound by the energy field of the nightshades.

The nightshade represents on a collective level a still existing dark age. Ignorance, arrogance, aggressiveness, fear of witches and demons, paired with escapism into dirty jokes and other cheap strategies.

Naturally not every Italian or southern European is like that. These are more or less a caricature of the complex personalities which exists in this country. There are a lot of exceptions. But you recognize the pattern. Movies depict them too as stereotypes, for which they are highly criticized. And homeopathic "character studies" are highly exaggerated in order to create a clear picture.

If you study miasms you will note collective themes. They require sometimes a nosode to break the cycle. According to Louis Klein, as he wrote in his excellent book "Miasms and Nosodes", if someone requires a nosode they believe that something is just not right with them. All nosodes have a parasitical characteristic. Interesting, because on this planet are a lot of parasites in human form.

CHAPTER SIX

Parasites

"Stay away from lazy parasites, who perch on you just
to satisfy their needs, they do not come to alleviate
your burdens, hence, their mission is to distract,
detract and extract, and make you live in abject
poverty."
(Michael Bassey Johnson)

One aspect of the plant family Anthemiaceae is described by Jan Scholten as "They are often abused by others. Others parasite on them, use their work and resources."

Artemisia cina, which makes part of this family, is well known as the "wormseed". The dried flowerheads are the source of the vermifugic drug santonin. As all Asteraceae they search for independency. From their point of view, independence does not mean to be free from all responsibility. It's more to be autonomous, to take one's own decisions. And they love to teach others to be autonomous too. One way to express this autonomy is to become a autodidact. Learning a lot and all by themselves what they need. Today this is possible for more people than in the past, thanks to books and tutorials on the internet.

A parasite search for a suitable host which provides enough resources. Capable people who have achieved a certain security and abundance, can be found in the Asteraceae family because of their ability to learn fast and on their own. They are ideal hosts for parasites. In order to not disturb them too much and risking to lose their host, parasites use subtle tricks to control their host.

Humans demonstrates evident psychic changes once they are infested by parasites. And parasites are not always insects, ticks or leeches. Human persons behave like parasites once they fall into a lower level of awareness. It's like they believe that they have the right to take forcibly what they need or want. I don't mean criminals, even if some of them are criminals or have a huge criminal potential. And not every criminal is like a parasite.

What I mean is that kind of person who acts exactly like a parasite. For example, which particular trait do we know from malaria? It is recurrent, right? A false friend is recurrent too. They will visit you and ask you for a big favour. They have this problem and only you, dear friend, can help them. And they know you will give them your money, because they have observed you, knowing that you are in this kind of situation where you are too weak to just say no.

Massimo Mangialavori analysed the common themes of parasites:
- egoism
- ambition
- growing

- greed
- alternating condition
- photophobia
- hunger
- cold
- meat

Or they try to exploit you in some other way. It happened to me once. I developed an online repertory for homeopathy based on the classic James Tyler Kent repertory. It attracted quit an attention in the world of homeopathy. Some doctors called me and asked if they can buy it. I said it's online and free for everyone. Just use it. Ah ok, well then, thanks. Another one, if I remember well he was a businessman from Austria, called me and asked if I was interested in a partnership. He would love to help me to promote the site. It would require some adjustments, a registering function for who wants to use a paid service, with some extra more data and so on. Well, ok, I was ready to accept his offer and asked him how to split the income, because I would do the bigger part of the work by programming all the stuff. He answered that unfortunately he already made a contract with another partner and they have split it fifty-fifty. I asked: "There is nothing for me, right?" He hesitated a bit and then came with this stupid argument, that he thought I would do all this because I love homeopathy. Sure, I love science, art, books, but I'm not an idiot to work for free for someone who just wants the maximum profit.

If you do experience this kind of parasitic attacks regularly, then ask yourself what attracts them. Is there a weakness inside yourself? Because parasites, doesn't matter if microorganisms or humans or even energetic entities, they can smell it.

In analysing the weakness, the simple repertorisation of physical symptoms can lead to the best result. A man got 3 symptoms, teeth grinding, itching anus and one very particular one, he saw small spots like lightnings.

Analysing it with Reference Works the result looks like this:

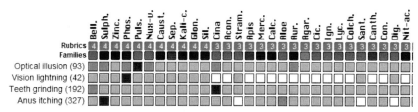

(MacRepertory ReferenceWorks)

Belladonna seems to be the remedy.

But it helped only partially. The 3 main symptoms remained as strong as before. Later the doctor decided to limit the analyses only on plants, because the patient's character seems to be complex and see what becomes visible.

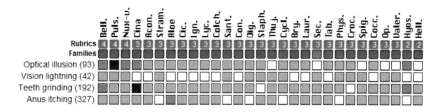

Now can you see the remedy which match better for this case? No? The doctor did know his patient well, he was a friend. He told him how often people tried to exploit him, asking money, favours, and so on. This is not a symptom you can repertorize. You need to know that the Asteraceae hate to be exploited and they get exploited quit often, more than other family groups. Finally, the doctor limited the family group on the Asterales.

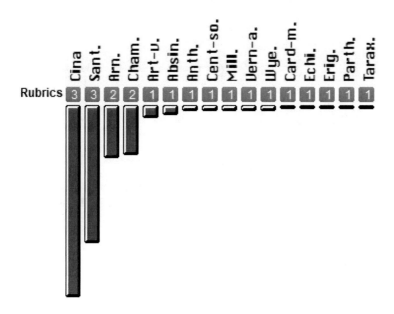

Artemisia cina came in front, followed by Santoninum which is the same remedy, only Cina is made of the whole plant and Santoninum are just the seeds.

Because his friend attracted so many "parasites" he gave him a CM10, which is a C10.000. The result was that his patient not only got better, but every human parasite flew from him. Now I ask you, how could the human parasites know that he would be able to repel them? They did not watch him in his eyes and recognize that now he was stronger and every attempt to exploit him would only result in a bold rejection. How could they tell that he was not a suitable host anymore?

In classical homeopathic literature we find a lot of cases where Cina in higher potencies helped children to get rid from intestinal worms. No need for toxic substances. The remedy changed the intestinal flora and the worms decided to leave. But in the case of human parasites, what changes? It's something deep in their consciousness, a shift in their energy level and awareness. It has nonlocal effects.

I would love to see a new rubric in repertories, with themes regarding such strange phenomenons. At the present time we need to translate such phenomenons into a symbolic language. When human parasites are attracted, a corresponding search for intestinal parasites in the repertory and materia medica is required.

CHAPTER SEVEN

Imponderabilia

"If you want to find the secrets of the universe, think
in terms of energy, frequency and vibration."
(Nikola Tesla)

Some manufacturers of homeopathic remedies may keep a distance from imponderabilia, because of their fear to appear not serious. I once wrote a critic about this, because I just don't get it why they are ok to produce homeopathic remedies, which are strange enough (nothing in it) or even sell Bach flower essences, and then refuse to sell imponderabilia remedies. Classic homeopaths like Hahnemann (who was more than "classic", he was the founder of homeopathy) wrote in his Organon §280 (the "bible of homeopathy") that "even imponderable agencies can produce most violent effects upon man".

What exactly are imponderabilia?

The original substance of homeopathic remedies are usually material substances, which you can touch, weight, smell and see. Imponderabilia are different. They have no mass and exist only at a vibrational, energetic level. For example, sunlight (Sol), moonlight (Luna), magnetism (The North or South pole of a magnet) and radiation (x-ray) are considered classic imponderabilia.

We overstep here the borders of the immaterial. It is certainly difficult to understand homeopathy per se, it becomes even more challenging for one to understand the imponderabilia. Materialists would hold their heads with their hands and refuse to continue to read. I'm so sorry for them. A worldview is like the lubrication oil of an engine. If one is unwilled to change it, the engine will get eventually a piston seizure. Then you can throw away the engine.

The immaterial is the real thing. Consciousness is the base of the material universe and of everything else beyond it. There is no doubt. But you need to make your own experiences, because it is not enough to read a book about dancing and then claim to have understood what dancing really is.

Symptoms produced by imponderabilia are more symbolic in their nature. Sure, they produce physical symptoms too. But the mind symptoms seem to transcendence every known limit. People who needs imponderabilia feels like there are no boundaries, no structure, no beginning and no end.

This reminds me of scientists who insists so much on the law of energy conservation, but then are not able to explain where the energy comes from for the electrons to fly endless around the proton core. They say "a perpetuum mobile" cannot exist. But if physical reality is based on consciousness, eternal principles could drive everything we know. It depends only on the interpretation of the universal mind. Eternity was there before time was created.

In the beginning (creation of time) God (universal mind and only true origin of consciousness) created heavens (space) and the earth (matter). We call the continuum inside physical reality the "spacetime". Time is bound to space on this level of reality. And space delivers boundaries. But there is a reality outside the physical reality, which existed before time itself. It is so abstract and difficult to understand, that a human who experienced just a blink of this realm would require decades to translate his experiences into a human language.

Imponderabilia represents this borders between the material and immaterial world. If DNA is considered a collection of words, then the meaning of the word is the imponderabilia, the immaterial, the idea.

Producing an imponderable remedy is such a strange process. For Sol, the sunlight, one concentrates the sun on globulis and then triturate them into C1, C2 and so on. Luna, the moonlight, is made in a similar process. A telescope collects the moonlight and concentrates them on the globulis.

As mentioned in chapter one, the intention of the laboratory assistant is the crucial factor. Globulis are always exposed to different radiation, sun, electromagnetism (cell phones, radar, wlan, galactic radiation from space ...), but when a imponderabilia is made, the morphic field of that specific source intended to be bound is linked to the lactose or carrier material and not all other billions of billions of different radiations surrounding it. The symptoms provoked by the proving of a remedy is proof enough.

People who get in resonance with imponderable energies have a problem to protect themselves and keep away from the boundaries between material and immaterial. Or maybe they channel this energy because the rest of the collective subconsciousness requires this energy. Like Nikola Tesla who received ideas and plans for his inventions, sometimes out of the blue like a lightning bolt, this people can possess the potential to change something big in the society. In contrast to Nux-moschata or Phosphorus, their connection to the immaterial world is real and exhibits power. But to be able to manage this power is not always possible if one has blockages which causes serious health problems. In this regard the imponderables are similar to the Actinides, which have huge potential power and are ready to explode if the energy is not constantly channelled and focused in a creative work. Vithoulkas definition of health states as follows:

> "... a good parameter for measuring the health of an individual is the degree to which he is free to create. Anybody who is basically healthy will seek to create rather than destroy. By creativity, as I have stated previously, I mean all those actions that promote the interests and good of oneself and others. To the degree that one commits destructive acts toward either himself or others, the degree to which he is diseased is apparent."
> (Prof. G. Vithoulkas)

To be "symptom free" is a rather dangerous way to define health, because a master of evil could be free from symptoms or a dead man could be free from symptoms, but not able to contribute in any way to the good of society.

Health implicates always the wellbeing of the individual and that of the collective of which the individual is a part. It promotes the unblocked and free stream of consciousness through all individuals, without restraints, energetic blockages or illusions or lies. It enhances the meaning of life and the happiness on short and long terms. Only a materialist loves to isolate and reduce elements into their parts, isolating them from their source and from the whole, denying the free will and denying that a meaning of life exists, ignoring higher complexity and interconnectedness. From this point of view materialism is a mental and spiritual illness.

Imponderabilia helps to stabilize the boundaries without closing the connection to this valuable source of energies. This is the case if an artist channels energy from planetary radiation, he could suffer from "burnout" syndrome because the amount of energy is just too much to handle at that time. The remedy removes the blockages which generates a kind of "friction", like electric resistors. Then the flow of energy becomes smooth and steady. Instead that the energy is received in phases and leaves the artist totally exhausted, the stream will be constant and remains open for the entire life. Without adequate help the organism could decide to close the stream for security reasons. And I'm afraid that the collective as a whole has closed the stream of life energy from the root source because of the one original lie. Else eternal life could be possible.

While you are reading this book, you may have noticed that I concentrate on the paradigm of an immaterial base of physical reality. Science is recognizing with some hesitation the fact that reality is in fact immaterial. Only our human perception makes it touchable. I admit that it was sometimes difficult to me to find a balance between the both worlds. They are not two realities in literal sense. There is only one reality, but different perceptions of it, which are called "worlds". The material aspect of the reality is condensed energy, linked in a loop until it becomes "dense", shared through all minds until it becomes a contract. Whoever needs a imponderabilia is able to feel that the material world is an illusion. But please let me clarify this word "illusion" in regard to the physical reality. Space and matter are necessary for us to experience the maximum closeness between individual minds, something for which angels envy us. Angels are complete creatures, genderless, no need for procreation, sleep, food, rest, and so on. But we humans are interlinked to each other human in the world-wide family, which is provided we are healthy a wonderful experience, unique, a continuing bliss. The imponderabilia represents the one extreme of this experience, when the awareness concentrates on the borders between matter and immaterial, between the dense and the "shen", the spirit. At the end what counts is balance.

CHAPTER EIGHT

Radionics

"And if everything within the physical realm is
powered by the same energy source, everything in
this realm is also bound to everything else through
this energy."
(Kelly Research Technologies)

"Radionics had an important influence on homeopathy and there are strong parallels between the two because many of the founders and practitioners of radionics were [and are] lay people e.g. George de la Warr, Malcolm Rae, Vernon Wethered, Jane Wilcox, Rosemary Russell, John Da Monte, Lavender Dower and Edith Eden. They also exerted an important influence from 1940-1970 upon the lay homeopathic movement because many of the figures involved were the same and mixed together. Also they shared the same remedies and often shared the same social scene. Homeopathy influenced radionics much more than the reverse, but nevertheless, they had a generally beneficial and benign influence on each other. Basically, radionics or radiesthesia depends very largely upon the dowsing faculty." (Hill, 1979, pp.161-9; Wethered, 1957, pp.13-63)

"They also shared the same dilemmas and difficulties and problems of being in a lay status and having the marginalisation and denigration from the medical majority allopaths. They also shared the same problems about tuition and passing on their skills to others of their kind." (Peter Morel, Radionic Homeopaths)

Hahnemann immaterialized the original substance by taking the raw original substance in a material form and freed it from its body (sal or salt in alchemy) by trituration or succussion, until the energy or blueprint was bound to the carrier material.

Radionics does the same thing, but more directly without even to use an original substance. It uses only the intention to get in touch with the energy of the plant or element or whatever one requires to balance an organism. Both radionics and homeopathy started on the material level, by experimenting with material substances and by advancing in their path they both recognized that going towards the immaterial has a deeper impact. For example, Hahnemann started with China in a material dose and then diluted and succussed it until the material part stepped into the background and the spirit of the original substance played its best performance. Almost the same happened to radionics. Dr. Albert Abrams discovery of radionics started with direct contact to the patient and ended with the earth as a medium. Other practitioners like Ruth Drown developed the technique further till to the point where diagnosis and treatment reached the point of "remote diagnosis and broadcasting".

Such awareness shift towards the immaterial for example happened to James Tyler Kent. Influenced by the teachings of Swedenborg Kent used higher and higher potencies. He was one of the first who set more emphasis on mind symptoms.

Radionics has many things in common with homeopathy. A radionics device looks like it has an electric function, emitting some sort of electromagnetic waves, or scalar-waves, bridging the gap of spacetime and achieving nonlocal influence on a remote organism. These devices are sold today for a few bucks till many thousands of dollars. Most of these devices has a label which warns the user to not open it. The reason is not only the loss of the guarantee, but the user would be baffled to see that it's a "black box" with no real function. There are a lot of LEDs blinking and it looks like an important technical device, decorating an alternative medicine therapist or doctor's office.

Radionics devices has just one function: they assist the operator in his intention. Nothing else.

"There's nothing in it" applies to radionics too!

I estimate that 99% of all radionics operators believe in a pseudoscientific theory. I admit that it's really difficult to accept that radionic devices are empty and has no real function, at least none in the physical realm, despite consuming electricity. But their design definitely is an aid to focus the intention of the operator over a longer period of time.

Somehow our mind needs help to ground and focus in order that the intention builds up enough potential to finish a work. During the dynamization process while creating homeopathic remedies the laboratory assistant performs a "ritual". The Organon the materia medica written by Hahnemann contains specific instruction for the dynamization of the remedies. Following these detailed rules, the intention of the operator will link the morphic field of the original substance to the carrier material, even if the operator has no clue how homeopathy works.

Similar a radionics operator does not need to be initiated in the secrets of how this art works. They just follow a set of instructions and the entire context focus their intention on the particular task. Advanced operators know that a radionics device works even if only painted as a circuit on a piece of paper.

April 2015 was an eye opener for me as it was almost exactly 20 years before. 1995 a friend of mine introduced me in homeopathy. I could not believe what he told me about this remedies with nothing in it. How could they possibly work? I was so sceptical about homeopathy that I decided to prove him wrong. In a library I read whatever I could find about homeopathy, it's founder Samuel Hahnemann and how remedies are made. Then I bought a high potency of Sulphur in a pharmacy and started a self-proving. The first dose before going to bed was miraculous. Vivid dreams full of yellow sceneries, an old locomotive and funny old men making jokes. When I woke up my blood came from my nose. Could it be a coincidence that I got these symptoms? I repeated the dose the next day. Again, very vivid dreams, and again blood from my nose and additionally fever. There was this itching on my skin and I perceived the odour of sulfur. I got ravenous hunger and a lot of other symptoms. Whenever I stopped taking the remedy the symptoms disappeared. They came back whenever I took it again. In order to be sure that the remedy was really just water and alcohol I diluted it further. Naturally not just simple dilution, but the dynamization process explained by Hahnemann, succussion and dilution. The higher potency revealed to be a lot stronger. My curiosity was awakened to its full extend. Now it was time to make my own remedy. The simplest approach was to make one of simple salt. In a book about homeopathy for beginners the author explained the process and I followed it step by step. I bought a mortar and milk sugar and triturated "common salt" (sodium chloride or $NaCl$) till to the C3 and then succussed it to the C30. During the trituration I got symptoms deriving undeniable from the essence of Natrium-muriaticum, which was strange because the amount of salt was minimal. You have more salt in a simple meal. But when I took the C30 the symptoms became unbearable. Sulfur was fun, but Natrium's essence feels so sad. I felt a lump in my throat and I was so weepy, that my brothers asked me what was wrong with me. This was proof enough for me. After that I started to study homeopathy and proved more than 40 different remedies during the last 20 years. Nobody can ever convince me that homeopathy does not work. I felt the effectiveness on myself.

And in April 2015, 20 years later, I read an article named "Homeodynamics, a window into the nature of reality", by Michael Leger on Interhomeopathy. The first few lines seemed ok, but then my eyes discovered the word "radionics" and my inner alarm went on. Leger explained that homeopathic remedies could be made with the help of a radionics device, without the original substance. I remembered what radionics was. Devices with nothing in it. Why did Interhomeopathy allow such a "muck" on a serious magazine, I thought at that time. As always, I needed to prove that it cannot work, unaware that history should repeat exactly as 20 years ago. I build a very simple radionics device myself, with the help of some electromagnetic coils which should produce "scalar waves", some LEDs, and a Arduino microprocessor with a software translating images into a sequence of light and em-pulses. This "information" was sent into blank globules (empty without a homeopathic information). As the "original substance" I took a self-made photo collage of LSD, the substance, its formula, and used that for the first self-made radionic remedy. History repeated. I took one dose and went to bed. After I closed my eyes I saw fractal patterns. Ok, I thought, this may be normal, because I tell myself that the remedy works. But the fractal patterns became stronger, more vivid, in full colour, in full resolution, higher than whatever I've seen before. My sense of time dissolved and I could not tell how long I was in that state. Then I slipped directly into a lucid dream, so vivid and clear. I remembered most the dream scenery from my childhood and some was unknown but very pleasant. Suddenly the scenery changed and it was not pleasant at all. Images of ergotism (Saint Anthony's Fire or ergot poisoning) dominated the dream, or nightmare. When I woke up I did a research on LSD and found out that this substance is similar to the Claviceps purpurea fungus, which contains a toxin similar to LSD, ergotamine. And LSD is known to provoke a high and a low, depending on the emotional setting before ingestion. I experienced both aspects of LSD, a high with pleasant feelings and imagery, but also a low. I did not expect a low in any way. So, radionics works, but why, why????

More experimentation followed. During the last 2 years my experience with radionics convinced me of the following, that it works because of the intention of the operator and only because of that. The radionics device helps to ground oneself and this is a kind of energetic protection, because using only your own intention without the device expose yourself to a variety of morphic fields. Also, the radionics device helps to focus. All the knobs and buttons and the rules and the rituals, these all help to concentrate and follow a routine which saves a lot of energy.

Does this mean now that homeopathic manufacturers will go bankrupt because everyone is able to produce their own remedy with a small device plugged into a USB-port of the computer?

I believe that this will not happen, because prior to this the global economic system will crash and never recover again.

But in fact, you can copy a homeopathic remedy by dynamizing it to the next potency. Just put one drop or one globule of the remedy in a new bottle with some water and alcohol and then shake it. Now you have a pirate copy, just as one is able to copy a software on a computer without paying for it. Fortunately, people don't do this (yet) and manufacturers of homeopathic remedies are respected, because they invest in research of new remedies too. Without them homeopathy would lose a big variety of high quality remedies, because dynamizing a remedy to a C1000 requires a lot of work (and focused intention). And I admit that there is indeed a difference between radionics made remedies and the classic homeopathic remedies you can buy in the pharmacy. Radionic remedies are more "soft" in their impact on the organism and don't act as long as homeopathic ones.

Radionics has a huge advantage in creating "new remedies" when the original substance is not available.

> The Homeodynamics method is particularly useful for the creation of remedies that are impossible by any other method. Human-based sarcodes, radioactive remedies from the actinide-series, and new nosodes are just three examples. Rather than using porcine or cadaver-based materials for sarcodes, we can directly reference the appropriate tissue, organ, etc. We can create remedies like neptunium carbonicum or something as exotic as einsteinium oxy-arsenicum. When a new organism has been identified, it can

also be developed into a remedy without exposing anyone to a potentially problematic situation.
(Michael Leger)

Michael Leger is right, there are remedies like for example Oganesson (symbol Og and atomic number 118). This element does not occur in nature and it can only be synthesized in laboratory. It's life span is very short. And even if a manufacturer can get his hands on a few milligrams, it would be very expensive and they would risk their lives because of the high radiation.

Radionics helps homeopathy to "synthesize" new or "exotic" remedies and represents the next level of homeopathy. I regard it as a "unleashed homeopathy", free from all boundaries of physical reality.

I plan to write a book on how to build your own radionics device, with step by step instruction, explaining the basics and some more advanced techniques, also how to install an open source software for radionics in your device.

But for now, I want to explain some more advanced possibilities of what is possible with radionics and homeopathy.

Copy a remedy
It is possible to copy a homeopathic remedy, just by putting the remedy bottle in the input well and another bottle with only water in the target well and activate the "copy function". After a few seconds the information is transmitted to the bottle in the target well.

Raise or lower the potency
A remedy in a C30 potency can be potentized to a higher or lower potency during the copy process. This is very convenient if one needs to fine tune a remedy to the right potency. Usually homeopaths use the standard C200, at least in Europe. But as in my case, I have a lot of remedies at home which are C1000 or higher. Now that I'm older a potency of more than C200 is too high for my organism. I react with stronger initial aggravations. This is totally normal and well known by experienced homeopaths. Now we don't need to buy new remedies in a lower potency. The radionics device helps to translate the potency to a lower one.

Dynamize a substance
A substance in raw state, or a tincture, can be dynamized in any potency too. This function is similar to the raising of the potency.

Combine raw substance with the dynamized energy
Globulis or water are used in homeopathy as carrier substances for the immaterial information or morphic field link.
With radionics we can use supplements pills instead and combine both with a stronger synergistic effect.

For example, St John's-wort could be combined with the homeopathic potency of Hypericum perforatum (Latin name for St John's wort), let's say a C12, plus some gem essence like "Smoky Quartz".

Such enhanced supplements pills could carry with them a "*program*" which prevents certain negative side effects. For example, St John's wort can provoke dentin hypersensitivity. A aetheric program could select from a list of acupuncture points the appropriate ones and gently stimulate them until the hypersensitivity is overcome or at least lessened. For more drastic side effects the program selects a remedy from a list of antidotes. In the case of St John's wort, the list includes: Ars., Cham. and Sulph.

Many supplements pills lack the energetic counterpart once the drug is dried. Radionics is able to recover the energetic field, make it stronger and more active.

Especially an illness which implies a severe malnutrition based on a malabsorption of the organism can be treated with this kind of approach. Remember please that in case of an illness a doctor should be consulted.

Homeopathic hair transmission
This is another odd way of using homeopathy. Dr. B. Sahni wrote a book called "*Transmission of homeopathic drug energy from a distance*". He mentions Dr. Abrams the inventor of radionics in the first few pages, then also Bovis and the old technique to measure energy with a pendulum. I regard Dr. Sahni as one of the most open-minded scientists. Inspired by Mr. Andre Simoneton technique to broadcast radionic pesticides over a distance with the use of

photographs, he rediscovered the treatment over distance by using homeopathic remedies applied to hair of the patient or a photograph. Dr. Sahni just use a photography of the patient and placed some globulis on top of it. The reaction was immediate, strong enough to provoke initial aggravations. His patients gave him feedback via telephone. Sometimes the reaction was too strong and he needed to remove the remedy from the photograph. He also tried to use hair or other "belongings" of the patients.

Now this may sound like magic, but Dr. Sahni is a doctor of medicine. Also, we should use logic to reason why this is possible. The framework of physical reality allows transmission of information of great distance because it is based on consciousness. Experiments with quantum entanglement proved that the distance does not matter. Information can be send faster than the speed of light, provided that an entanglement between the sender and receiver exist. Well we breath all the same air, therefore we can assume that this entanglement between all human on this planet must exist. If our creator has created everything in a way which allows this kind of communication, there must exist a good reason why it is possible. Nonlocal communication between plants has proved to be live saving. Experiments with a lie detector attached to plants showed that a plant hurt intentionally by an experimenter results in peaks in the polygraph attached to other plants placed in distant rooms or even in other buildings. These experiments were conducted the first time by Grover Cleveland "Cleve" Backster, Jr., an interrogation specialist for the CIA. On Wikipedia an article says that plant perception or biocommunication is the idea that plants are sentient, that they respond to humans in a manner that amounts to ESP, and that they experience pain and fear. Now even ants and termites seem to communicate over big distances. This assures their survival. For example, the nuptial flight of many colonies is synchronized at the same time. Birds loves these events, because they catch the ants in the flight as uninvited partakers of the wedding breakfast. If only one colony at the time would initiate the nuptial flight, the risk that most of the ants would be eaten by the birds is too high. But many colonies start their wedding at the same time. This occurs in such a synchronous manner, that the birds cannot concentrate on just one colony.

Another example of nonlocality and synchronicity which enables our survival is photosynthesis! Quantum biologists' studies how photons are distributed inside a plant leaf. Once the photon enters the leaf it is still in the form of a wave. This wave is a probability wave, which means it is not located yet. Indeed, it exists everywhere in the universe at the same time, but there is a higher chance that it will collapse as a particle inside the leaf and by this release its energy to the chlorophyll unit which is in the biggest need of energy for producing nutriment for the plant and as a byproduct oxygen. If we study nature, especially in the quantum biology field, nonlocality and synchronicity reveals to be crucial for life. It is essential, no doubt.

It may seem to be so strange if a doctor places the homeopathic remedy on the photograph or the hair of the patient and then the patient feels the effect and gets better. But here is no magic involved.

I was 8 years old when I asked our catholic priest in our town what the difference is between the wonders performed by Jesus Christ and magic practice. This question was like a burning fire in me waiting to leave my mouth, because back then I just could not see any difference. The priest was assigned to us as a substitution for our religion teacher in Germany. He looked at me in a despising manner and said in front of the entire class: „You are too stupid to understand!" (in German: "Du bist zu dumm um das zu verstehen!"). Man, I felt so much hate for this old man! Later I decided to leave the church. Besides the hypocrisy of the priest and the whole organization, I was absolutely unsatisfied with their teaching and dogmatism. Ten years later I unregistered from this religion and began my search for the truth. Whatever you want to know about God is written in the Bible, the only book which tells you the whole truth. Even Nikola Tesla wrote in his autobiography that everyone should read this book.

> The gift of mental power comes from God, Divine Being, and if we concentrate our minds on that truth, we become in tune with this great power. My Mother had taught me to seek all truth in the Bible; therefore I devoted the next few months to the study of this work.
> (Nikola Tesla)

In Galatians 5:19-21 witchcraft is mentioned together with other bad things like hostility, strife, jealousy, fits of anger and so on. In the light of this scripture, how can the teleportation of a healing information by the mean of the use of nonlocal phenomenons regarded as magic, if the intention of the doctor is benevolent? The transmission of the homeopathic drug occurs with the consent of the patient. Alternatively, the doctor could have used the telephone to tell his patient that he needs a specific remedy and to buy it in his local pharmacy. But the transmission of the "name of the remedy" via phone would be regarded as "magic" in ancient times by people who was ignorant regarding modern technology.

> When a distinguished but elderly scientist states that something is possible, they are almost certainly right. When they state that something is impossible, they are very probably wrong.

> The only way of discovering the limits of the possible is to venture a little way past them into the impossible.

> Any sufficiently advanced technology is indistinguishable from magic.

> (Arthur C. Clarke)

Only the intention to subdue the free will of someone else to its own will can be regarded as magic, because this is indeed the modern definition of magic practice. In this regard there is no difference between lies, corruption and illusions. In 1 Samuel 15:23 we can read that pushing ahead presumptuously is the same as using magical power and idolatry. Here it is made clear, that the intention counts. You can use a cell phone to remotely contact another person. This is not magic. But if you tell the other person on the other side a lie with the intention to harm, then there is no difference between magic or "pushing ahead presumptuously". Magic is just a word describing the practice of an ancient religious caste of the Medes (the Magi) who misused "natural" phenomenons such as nonlocal transmission for their criminal acts. Naturally all phenomenons of nature can be misused, as every technology too. In our modern time, since 1914, technology is the main aspect in warfare and it is more powerful than every known magic practice. Nuclear rockets can reach a country in a few minutes and burn the earth on the ground of a city with such a high temperature that it transforms into glass. It is always the intention what counts.

CHAPTER NINE

Teleportation of DNA

"Beam me up, Scotty"
(Captain Kirk)

What exactly is the function of DNA in a biological organism? Science textbooks for school says it contains build plans for the body (or plant), where everything is described in minuscule details. A classic example is the colour of the iris, which is written inside the DNA. The truth is not so simple. DNA contains information for the synthesis of many building blocks like proteins, also for hormones and enzymes, but no information was ever encoded which points towards the building plan of the form of organs and the entire body. Strangely the DNA seems to lack information about the form and formative processes. This was one of the main research goals of Dr. Rupert Sheldrake. The information of the form is elsewhere, immaterial and invisible.

Imagine this scenario. You are a construction worker. At the construction site trucks delivers the raw material for making the bricks, clay, water, and so on. Together with the clay you receive the building plan for the bricks, the specific form of the bricks only. And you may wonder where the plan for the house is. Well, the entire plan for the house is send to you via email, wireless, broadcasted through the aether. Your computer is able to interpret the electromagnetic vibrations and then displays the blueprint of the house on the display. In order to be able to receive the information it needs an antenna calibrated on a specific frequency.

In a similar way this applies to the DNA too. But it is a little bit more complex than a simple computer build by human beings. The DNA is a vibrant construct in itself, able to adjust itself to different frequencies. I get goose bumps when I think about the DNA. It's a chain of harmonic oscillators with dipole-dipole interaction between nearest neighbours resulting in a van der Waals type bonding. The entire structure remains only stable because it generates a standing wave and the binding energy is quantum entanglement. It is like an instrument is made of the music it should play!!! How can this ever have evolved from a *"primeval soup"*? Only a super intelligent being could have designed this kind of technology. The DNA is a dynamic antenna receiving and broadcasting information towards a *"biological internet"*. To call it just a library of information is an oversimplification and misleading.

The case Jacques Benveniste
1988 Jacques Benveniste published a controversial paper in the scientific journal Nature. He described how high dilutions of

antibody proteins in water was still biologically active, which support the concept of homeopathy. Benveniste concluded that water molecule configurations are responsible for the "*memory of water*". This water molecule clusters are able to memorize the electromagnetic signature of the original substance and to transmit it to biological cells. Later in the nineties Benveniste asserted that this "*memory*" could be digitized, transmitted and reinserted into another sample of water, which would exhibit similar biological activity on organisms or cells.

As usual dogmatism was the incentive for certain people who proposed a follow-up investigation. Nature send a team put together with non-scientists, aka one well-known self-professed skeptic James Randi, a so called "*fraud expert*" Walter Stewart and John Maddox himself, the editor of Nature. It was Benveniste who invited the team of Nature to design their own double-blind procedure and so they did. The results were negative. Strange, because after this incident several independent laboratories was successful in reproducing Benveniste's experiment. One of the scientists who replicated it was no one less than Luc Antoine Montagnier, Nobel Prize winner in medicine for his discovery of the HIV virus.

I guess that the only difference between success and failure was the absence of an inhibiting factor, skepticism and the intention to see failure at all costs. At a certain level the observer becomes part of the experiment. People like James Randi exhibits a similar effect on the experiment like Wolfgang Pauli did back in his days. For example, according to some anecdotes whenever Pauli entered a laboratory room experiments failed or machinery broke down. Even Pauli believed in it. Some of his friends working at the lab wouldn't allow him to visit them there anymore. This can be regarded as superstition, but they were all scientists. Eventually you just cannot deny the fact of frequent synchronistic events. In my opinion James Randi should be banned from this kind of experiments. Just a suggestion. Don't take it too seriously.

Teleporting DNA over the Internet
In March 2009 it was Montagnier's turn. He published a paper titled "*Electromagnetic signals are produced by aqueous nanostructures derived from bacterial DNA sequences*". The electromagnetic signals of Escherichia coli bacteria were recorded and digitized in form of a waveform audio file (*.wav). This electrical signature was

then send to a distant pure water sample, where DNA can replicate through PCR (polymerase chain reaction) despite the absence of the original DNA.

How does "*DNA teleportation*" work?

Marc Henry, a scientist of the University of Strasbourg, explains what happens on quantum scale: liquid water molecules tend to "*hold hands with each other*", which is known as hydrogen bond. At a certain point they form a closed space where matter cannot get in. However, everything electromagnetic can get in. All these signals can be trapped inside the space, what is called a coherent domain.

The coherent oscillations of electron clouds in water molecules are the cause and consequence at the same time. What Montagnier's experiment involves is to record the signals from this electron cloud inside the water cluster. This becomes only possible once the DNA was diluted and potentised till the D6 or D7 potency. At this potency the water emits the strongest signal in a frequency range of 20 to 20.000 Hz, which is super interesting, because this is also the same range the human ear can hear. In some way the DNA's own electromagnetic signal is trapped in a temporary sphere of water molecules and by dilution the DNA get lost, but not the signal. Now the water is playing a music which resembles the structure of the original DNA.

Till now even a materialistic scientist is able to follow and to understand why water has a memory. But the experiment reaches a peak of craziness where a materialistic worldview cannot withstand and must crumble.

The signal is recorded and send by email to another laboratory, in Italy Benevento, to the University of Sannio known for their specialization in molecular biology. There Vittorio Colantuoni and Giuseppe Vitello treat a sample of pure water for one hour with the "*music of the DNA*". After that they put the water in a PCR chamber, with isolated nucleotides and a DNA primer. The polymerase chain reaction is used normally to clone a particular DNA sequence, with a physical present DNA strand. But the experiment now involves only pure water with an electromagnetic signal trapped in water clusters. A signal which is only few kilobytes big.

In order to reproduce a complete DNA sequence, you will need 600MB of data. This data fills a CD-ROM almost completely. Do you remember the 3,5-inch diskettes? You need 417 floppy disks to memorize this amount of data, with a weight of 7 kilogram (16 pounds)! And you cannot transmit this amount of data via email (not in 2018). Watching closely film material about the experiment of Montagnier you can see clearly that the file must be very small, because the wav sample is only few seconds long and they play it in repeat mode for one hour. So how is it possible that a DNA of a size of several hundreds of megabytes can be compressed in only few kilobytes? It's not possible with any mathematical compressing algorithm. But here comes the idealistic worldview in play. If the signal represents a key and not the entire sequence, then it makes sense. A key is like a symbol. Everyone knows what the symbol of a snake means, or red colour, or a triangle. The collective consciousness is able to interpret the symbol and act accordingly. On the quantum level the polymerase chain reaction retrieves the information of the entire DNA sequence just from the key signal of a few kilobytes and rebuilds an almost complete copy of the original DNA. Montagnier said in an interview that the replication experiments conducted in Germany and Italy reproduced a DNA sequence identical to 98%. This is more than enough evidence.

Giuseppe Vitello from the University of Benevento said, that the experiment is quite simple and beautiful and that he feels *young again, like when I started making research*. Dogmatism is a frustrating way to think and it's the desperate attempt to hold progress back. Vittorio Colantuoni was amazed by the results and he admits that the experiment is a turning point in biology, physics and knowledge too. Also, he can understand why there are so many skepticals. Montagnier said that this experiment makes a lot of people grinding their teeth.

Max Planck once said that truth never triumphs. Its opponents just die out. Science advances one funeral at a time. He was right. Dogmatism can be regarded as a *spiritual illness* for which really no cure exists rather than death. This illness is rooted in the deepest level of a dogmatic person, based on their very motivations. You can never ever convince such a person from the contrary, because the implication of the knowledge is contradictory to their imagination and their will. They hate you for not sustaining their consensus reality, for not playing their game.

CHAPTER TEN

DNA Phantom Effect

"Nature abhors a vacuum"
(Aristotle)

10 years before Montagnier's experiment with DNA teleportation another experiment made it to the top of the high score of fringe science.

Dr. Poponin, a quantum biologist from Russia, specialized in nonlinear dynamics of DNA and the interactions of weak electromagnetic fields with biological systems, made a discovery about *"empty space"* and DNA.

Inside a temperature controlled *"scattering chamber"* a DNA sample is placed. A laser shoot photons concentrated with the help of a collimator. The photons reflected by the DNA strand are then again redirected with another collimator into a photon multiplier. At the end a photon counter and a correlation analyser are fed with the photons. The autocorrelation function shows a significant pattern, similar to a shape of an oscillatory and slowly exponentially decaying function. Now the fascinating aspect reveals when the experimenters removed the DNA from the chamber. Instead of showing the same chaotic background noise before the DNA was placed into the chamber, the autocorrelation function shows now a similar oscillatory pattern. And these patterns remain for an extended period of time, as if it is attached to the space inside the chamber.

If the experimenter repeats the measurement, after say one day or two, the oscillatory pattern changes in its frequency. Than more time pass, than higher the frequency becomes, eventually so high that no measurement device made by humans is able to measure it.

Where did the information of the DNA go?
There is a theory called *"scalar waves"* which explains that a electromagnetic wave is able to leave spacetime and travel only on the timeline. Every typical aspect of spacetime like decay and entropy does not have an effect on the timeline. The information travelling on this one dimension only is at the same time *"everywhere"*, because time is everywhere. Indeed, the scalar wave theory is much older than quantum mechanics, but it has so many similarities. I regard both theories as complementary, pointing towards a bigger picture. At a certain point the mind does not care about the space relationship, but it concentrates only on the evolving aspect on the timeline. The nonlocal quantum wave, which travels on the timeline, collapses if an observer wants to know where

the particle is. Only then the energy is released into spacetime, only if it makes "*sense*". Then the information on the timeline gets in touch with space and "*relates*" again with matter. The DNA phantom experiment is proof of the ability of the entire framework we call reality to persist memory without any decay or loss.

That fact that memory is a intrinsic part of spacetime is a painful thorn in the eyes of materialists. They hate this phenomenons, because it reveals the failure of their oversimplified worldview. They did everything possible to remove this aspect from their science books. They call empty space "*vacuum*" and they hoped to be able to replace the "*aether*" theory. In the past the aether was considered as a medium, with characteristics similar to air. And indeed, the aether theory is more accurate that the vacuum theory, because there is no real empty space. Even ultra-high vacuum contains 100 particles/cm3 and this a lot, because every atom has a electromagnetic field surrounding the nucleus, so big that it will fill without problem the entire cm3 of space. Most alternative science researcher (or fringe scientists) believe in the aether and not in an empty space called vacuum. They have used their own vocabulary, like Wilhelm Reich's orgone, but most time they pointed towards an aether acting as a medium between the particles. Wilhelm Reich was one of the most suppressed scientists of all time. If you study science history by keeping in mind that censorship and suppression exerted by materialists is everywhere and a constant factor, you will recognize how much frustration and pain they have caused throughout many centuries of "*modern times*". No wonder why so many fringe scientists decides to keep hidden in the shadows or to publish their work under a pseudonym. But there will be better times.

Modern science books should teach according to the first verse of Genesis. "*In the beginning (time) God (most supreme consciousness) created heavens (space) and earth (matter).*" According to this verse from the Bible a science book of 1000 pages should teach 250 pages on the phenomenon of time only, another 250 pages on consciousness, 250 on space and then the remaining 250 on matter. If you take a modern book on general physics today it's about 99% about matter, because we live in a materialistic world. The ideal science book would explain the nonlocal, the timeless or eternal and the time, how it relates to consciousness and then, only after that it would explain spacetime and matter. In such a perfect science book phenomenons like DNA teleportation and DNA phantom effect would be mentioned in the opening chapter for matter, even before chemistry is mentioned. I'm looking forward to read such a book in the future.

CHAPTER ELEVEN

Hahnemann and Mesmerism

"A responsive influence exists between the heavenly
bodies, the earth, and animated bodies."
(Franz Anton Mesmer)

Every homeopath I met got at least a copy of the Organon, the most important book in homeopathy written by Samuel Hahnemann. To be specific, every one of them got at least the fifth edition. In these editions Hahnemann included additional aphorisms about Franz Anton Mesmer in the paragraphs 293 to 294 (288 in the sixth edition). Every homeopath claimed to have read the entire Organon, but none of them remembered these aphorisms about animal magnetism mentioned by Hahnemann, which is strange, but a normal phenomenon, because you only remember what you are able to integrate into your worldview. Indeed, Hahnemann gave specific instructions how to use this phenomenon in difficult cases, when the life force was too weak to react to a homeopathic stimulus, or in cases when the life force was confused by too many remedies given in a short period of time.

Samuel Hahnemann recognized some truth in Franz Anton Mesmer teaching regarding this life force phenomena. Mesmer's described in his "Propositions Concerning Animal Magnetism" from 1779:

1. A responsive influence exists between the heavenly bodies, the earth, and animated bodies.
2. A fluid universally diffused, so continuous as not to admit of a vacuum, incomparably subtle, and naturally susceptible of receiving, propagating, and communicating all motor disturbances, is the means of this influence.
3. This reciprocal action is subject to mechanical laws, with which we are not as yet acquainted.
4. Alternative effects result from this action, which may be considered to be a flux and reflux.
5. This reflux is more or less general, more or less special, more or less compound, according to the nature of the causes which determine it.
6. It is by this action, the most universal which occurs in nature, that the exercise of active relations takes place between the heavenly bodies, the earth, and its constituent parts.
7. The properties of matter and of organic substance depend on this action.
8. The animal body experiences the alternative effects of this agent and is directly affected by its insinuation into the substance of the nerves.

9. Properties are displayed, analogous to those of the magnet, particularly in the human body, in which diverse and opposite poles are likewise to be distinguished, and these may be communicated, changed, destroyed, and reinforced.

10. Even the phenomenon of declination may be observed.

11. This property of the human body which renders it susceptible of the influence of heavenly bodies, and of the reciprocal action of those which environ it, manifests its analogy with the magnet, and this has decided me to adopt the term of animal magnetism

12. The action and virtue of animal magnetism, thus characterized, may be communicated to other animate or inanimate bodies. Both of these classes of bodies, however, vary in their susceptibility.

13. Experiments show that there is a diffusion of matter, subtle enough to penetrate all bodies without any considerable loss of energy.

14. This action and virtue may be strengthened and diffused by such bodies.

15. Its action takes place at a remote distance, without the aid of any intermediary substance.

16. It is, like light, increased and reflected by mirrors.

17. It is communicated, propagated, and increased by sound.

18. This magnetic virtue may be accumulated, concentrated, and transported.

19. I have said that animated bodies are not all equally susceptible; in a few instances they have such an opposite property that their presence is enough to destroy all the effects of magnetism upon other bodies.

20. This opposite virtue likewise penetrates all bodies: it also may be communicated, propagated, accumulated, concentrated, and transported, reflected by mirrors, and propagated by sound. This does not merely constitute a negative, but a positive opposite virtue.

21. The magnet, whether natural or artificial, is like other bodies susceptible of animal magnetism, and even of the opposite virtue: in neither case does its action on fire and the needle [of a compass] suffer any change, and this shows that the principle of animal magnetism essentially differs from that of mineral magnetism.

22. This system sheds new light upon the nature of fire and of light, as well as on the theory of attraction, of flux and reflux, of the magnet and of electricity.

23. It teaches us that the magnet and artificial electricity have, with respect to diseases, properties common to a host of other agents presented to us by nature, and that if the use of these has been attended by some useful results, they are due to animal magnetism.

24. These facts show, in accordance with the practical rules I am about to establish, that this principle will cure nervous diseases directly, and other diseases indirectly. By its aid the physician is enlightened as to the use of medicine, and may render its action more perfect, and can provoke and direct salutary crises, so as to completely control them.

25. In communicating my method, I shall, by a new theory of matter, demonstrate the universal utility of the principle I seek to establish.

26. Possessed of this knowledge, the physician may judge with certainty of the origin, nature, and progress of diseases, however complicated they may be; he may hinder their development and accomplish their cure without exposing the patient to dangerous and troublesome consequences, irrespective of age, temperament, and sex. Even women in a state of pregnancy, and during parturition, may reap the same advantage.

27. This doctrine will finally enable the physician to decide upon the health of every individual, and of the presence of the diseases to which he may be exposed. In this way the art of healing may be brought to absolute perfection.

Sure, Mesmer's terminology was not that of a quantum physicist, but he made accurate observations and this is in the end what really counts.

Hahnemann understood that this life force was indeed the reacting force to the homeopathic remedies. What follows are the two paragraphs from the fifth edition.

§293
I find it necessary to allude here to animal magnetism, as it is termed, or rather mesmerism (as it should be called, out of gratitude to Mesmer, its first founder), which differs so much in its nature from all other therapeutic agents. This curative power, often so stupidly denied, which streams upon a patient by the contact of a well-intentioned person powerfully

exerting his will, either acts homoeopathically, by the
production of symptoms similar to those of the diseased state
to be cured; and for this purpose a single pass made, without
much exertion of the will, with the palms of the hands not too
slowly from the top of the head downwards over the body to
the tips of the toes,[1] is serviceable in, for instance, uterine
hemorrhages, even in the last stage when death seems
approaching; or it is useful by distributing the vital force
uniformly throughout the organism, when it is in abnormal
excess in one part and deficient in other parts, for example, in
rush of blood to the head and sleepless, anxious restlessness
of weakly persons, etc., by means of a similar, single, but
somewhat stronger pass; or for the immediate
communication and restoration of the vital force to some one
weakened part or to the whole organism, - an object that
cannot be attained so certainly and with so little interference
with the other medicinal treatment by any other agent besides
mesmerism. If it is wished to supply a particular part with the
vital force, this is effected by concentrating a very powerful
and well-intentioned will for the purpose, and placing the
hands or tips of the fingers on the chronically weakened parts,
whither an internal chronic dyscrasia has transferred its
important local symptom, as, for example, in the case of old
ulcers, amaurosis, paralysis of certain limbs, etc.[2] Many
rapid apparent cures performed in all ages, by mesmerizers
endowed with great natural power, belong to this class. The
effect of communicated human power upon the whole human
organism was most brilliantly shown, in the resuscitation of
persons who had lain some time apparently dead, by the most
powerful sympathetic will of a man in full vigor of vital
force,[3] and of this kind of resurrection history records many
undeniable examples.

1. The smallest homoeopathic dose, which however,
   often effects wonders when used on proper occasions.
   Imperfect homoeopaths, who think themselves
   monstrously clever, not infrequently deluge their
   patients in difficult diseases with doses of different
   medicines, given rapidly one after the other, which,
   although they may have been homoeopathically
   selected and given in highly potentized attenuation,
   bring the patients into such an over-excited state that

life and death are struggling for the mastery, and the least additional quantity of medicine would infallibly kill them. In such cases a mere gentle mesmeric pass and the frequent application, for a short time of the hand of a well-intentioned person to the part that is particularly affected, produce the harmonious uniform distribution of the vital force throughout the organism, and therewith rest, sleep and recovery.

2. Although by this restoration of the vital force, which ought to be repeated from time to time, no permanent cure can be affected in cases where, as has been taught above, a general internal dyscrasia lies at the root of the old local affection, as it always does, yet this positive strengthening and immediate saturation with the vital force (which no more belongs to the category of palliatives than does eating and drinking when hunger and thirst are present) is no mean auxiliary to the actual treatment of the whole disease by homoeopathic   medicines.

3. Especially of one of those persons, of whom there are not many who, along with great kindness of disposition and perfect bodily powers, possesses but a very moderate desire for sexual intercourse, which it would give him very little trouble to suppress, in whom, consequently, all the fine vital spirits that would otherwise be employed in the preparation of the semen, are ready to be communicated to others, by touching them and powerfully exerting the will. Some powerful mesmerisers, with whom I have become acquainted, has all this peculiar character.

§294
All the above-mentioned methods of practicing mesmerism depend upon an influx of more or less vital force into the patient, and hence are termed positive mesmerism.[1] An opposite mode of employing mesmerism, however, as it produces just the contrary effect, deserves to be termed negative mesmerism. To this belong the passes which are used to rouse from the somnambulic sleep, as also all the manual processes known by the names of soothing and ventilating.

This discharge by means of negative mesmerism of the vital force accumulated to excess in individual parts of the system of debilitated persons is most surely and simply performed by making a very rapid motion of the flat extended hand, held parallel to, and about an inch distant from the body, from the top of the head to the tips of the toes.[2] The more rapidly this pass is made, so much the more effectually will the discharge be affected. Thus, for instance, in the case where a previously healthy woman,[3] from the sudden suppression of her catamenia by a violent mental shock, lies to all appearance dead, the vital force which is probably accumulated in the precordial region, will by such a rapid negative pass, be discharged and its equilibrium throughout the whole organism restored, so that the resuscitation generally follows immediately.[4] In like manner, a gentle, less rapid, negative pass diminishes the excessive restlessness and sleeplessness accompanied with anxiety sometimes produced in very irritable persons by a too powerful positive pass, etc.

1. When I here speak of the decided and certain curative power of positive mesmerism, I most assuredly do not mean the abuse of it, where, by repeated passes of this kind, continued for half an hour or a whole hour at a time, and, even day after day, performed on weak, nervous patients, that monstrous revolution of the whole human system is affected which is termed somnambulism, wherein the human being is ravished from the world of sense and seems to belong more to the world of spirits - a highly unnatural and dangerous state, by means of which it has not infrequently been attempted to cure chronic diseases.

2. It is a well known rule that a person who is either to be positively or negatively mesmerised, should not wear silk on any part of the body.

3. Hence a negative pass, especially if it be very rapid, is extremely injurious to a delicate person affected with a chronic ailment and deficient in vital force.

> 4.   A strong country lad, ten years of age, received in the morning, on account of slight indisposition, from a professed female mesmeriser, several very powerful passes with the points of both thumbs, from the pit of the stomach along the lower edge of the ribs, and he instantly grew pale, and fell into such a state of unconsciousness and immobility that no effort could arouse him, and he was almost given up for dead. I made his eldest brother give him a very rapid negative pass from the crown of the head over the body to the feet, and in one instant he recovered his consciousness and became lively and well.

Hahnemann and contemporaries of him like Mesmer described a phenomenon already known from other therapy systems like acupuncture. If you have studied TCM (Traditional Chinese Medicine) you will recognize a lot of similarities in Mesmers teaching and in Hahnemann's observation written in his §293 to 294. For example, what Mesmer wrote *"A responsive influence exists between the heavenly bodies, the earth, and animated bodies"* is taught also by the QiGong masters today. During their advanced training their life force gets in resonance with their surroundings and a deep balanced state can be reached. Their awareness for the inner flow of energy as also of their surroundings is enhanced.

Also *"alternative effects result from this action, which may be considered to be a flux and reflux"* points towards a energy flow which obeys certain laws. Wilhelm Reich too observed independently some decades later this flow in humans as also in the nature. For example, the weather is generated by this kind of energy flows in the atmosphere. Severe drought periods in deserts are mostly caused by stuck energy, blockages in the earth's and atmosphere's energy channel. Wilhelm Reich believed that these can be healed and by doing so the weather would change in these areas. He demonstrated that on different occasions when he brought back rain in desertic areas.

Hahnemann description of this phenomena are coherent with the QiGong theory. He wrote that *"a well-intentioned person powerfully exerting his will"* and *"concentrating a very powerful and well-intentioned will for the purpose"*, pointing towards a similar description in many QiGong literature, that the will-power (yi) and intention is what is able to lead and control the Qi, the life force.

If you study TCM, especially the *"inner arts"* of NeiDan or NeiKung, you will always be reminded that an abundance of Qi can only be generated by abstinence of sexual intercourse (not to mention the huge damage pornography and masturbation can do to the mind, the willpower and energy channels of a human being). The loss of semen needs to be avoided at all costs if one wants to use his life force for such a healing purpose. Not only that, but one needs to be able to transform (transmute) the force of a lower quality (jing), which would otherwise be utilized to generate semen, into a higher form of Qi, which is called Shen.

Read again the description of Hahnemann of what kind of person is required to practice this kind of energy work (italics and underlines are now mine):

> Especially of one of those persons, of whom there are not many who, along with *great kindness* of disposition and *perfect bodily powers*, possesses but <u>a *very moderate desire for sexual intercourse*, which it would give him very little trouble to suppress, in whom, consequently, *all the fine vital spirits that would otherwise be employed in the preparation of the semen, are ready to be communicated to others*</u>, by *touching* them and *powerfully exerting the will*. Some powerful mesmerisers, with whom I have become acquainted, has all this peculiar character.

Hahnemann's keen ability of observation lead him once again to recognize another truth, that the transmutation of "semen" into higher vibrational energies not only requires the simple abstinence, but an inner attitude which would not require at all a suppressing of the desire for sexual intercourse, because as many others like Wilhelm Reich observed, a suppression leads to more blockages and eventually to a lower energy level. This kind of abstinence should derive from a natural inclination, free will and a deep conviction. And as Hahnemann wrote *"there are not many"* of them. Instead the situation today is worse: Young men waste their semen for nothing, like smokers addicted to tobacco waste their money for nothing, just smoke and dirty smelly air.

CHAPTER TWELVE

Mind over Matter

"It's all mind over matter.
If I don't mind, it doesn't matter."

A universe created by a superior mind, based solely on the immaterial consciousness, stable and coherent from the microcosms till to the macrocosms, enabling life for billions of individuals who enjoy a free will, ... put in a discordant element and observe how the system reacts to rebalance itself. You can observe this when you make a homeopathic proving, when you get symptoms from the remedy, when you feel that something is not right and that the reaction is there to make it all a whole image again.

Our mind is able to provoke phenomenons like the "*stigmata*", when blood comes out of the middle of the palm of the hand, out of the "*laogong*" acupuncture point (PC-8), by overheating the pericardium meridian and driving the blood out of the hand. This is mind over matter, it works because the mind is the base of the universe and not the other way around. Would the universe be based on pure matter, then there would be no mind as such and no free will at all?

Things goes wrong when inside the individual mind a lie or illusion persist. If this lie is evaluated and determined as a truth, then it leads to perversion of what is natural. Think about it, if a person comes into the state of Stramonium Datura and he believes that every other human is his enemy, how will he consider his neighbour? This over agitated state of mind is not natural. A human being is not a plant, he is not Stramonium, but simply a human being. But the illusion, maybe triggered by an external source like a trauma, infiltrates inside his mind a wrong picture of himself and his surroundings. Now he thinks and acts like a lower being, a plant, an animal or a chemical element. The result is the production of symptoms, which are mirrors of the inner state of mind and soul.

This new state of mind lacks always the freedom which derives of human's full ability to exert their free will without any interference of an inner source of discordance. But it will mirror now the dissonant frequency on the matter, the body, it's functions and processes. It is still able to exhibits mind over matter force, as long as the human being is alive and breaths.

I believe that a perfect human being has extraordinary abilities, which are regarded today as paranormal abilities. This means such a perfect human could exhibit his will to control the weather, to transmute elements from one into another, to imprint mental images into crystals like a programmer writes software, and so many more phenomenons. The normal natural state of a human being is not decay and death, and we need to admit it, we feel that death is unnatural.

And yes, death is the end of the free will, when the mind reaches the lower end of the material state, when the harmony and interdependency becomes chaos and independence. Why should a nation celebrate "Independence Day" every year on the same day, if this in reality means the loss of liberty? The independence from God is the "*new normal*" since the adoption of a lie and this means the independence from the source of life. But the abundance of symptoms which are generated cannot be suppressed enough by the pharma industry. It will always be clear what is inside our imperfect mind, what is still wrong. Our body does not lie.

On planetary scale the weather changes and frequency of earthquakes increase permanently. There is no harmony between heaven and earth. Something subtler than the human mind interferes with the energy channels inside the earth and the cosmos. This leads to instability of the elements and tension is build up. So, there is not a free flow of energy from heaven to earth, but a tension prevents this flow. The tension is released in an uncontrolled manner by the earthquakes or by hurricanes.

Homeopathy for sure has its limitation regarding human's core problems. If someone search for help and visits a homeopath, they already decided to do something against their illness. They recognize that they are indeed ill. But real evil is not even not aware of their illness, but they desire perversion. Which remedy could ever reverse their decision to do what is wrong? There is no hope for the evil, no cure at all. It can only be removed from existence. And this requires divine intervention. When this happens, and it may happen very soon, the signs in heaven will be visible to everyone. When God exhibits his will over the earth, no human made weapon can protect the nations against his wrath. The phenomena of "*Mind over matter*" will reach the highest levels of impact when the very source of the mind is angelical. In the end the imbalance will be removed, the dissonance ceases to exist and perfect health is not anymore, a tail from utopia. Millions of people put their faith in this hope. What can an imperfect human being do compare to this army of heaven? We are able to do extraordinary things, yes we can, but we have limits and we would be the biggest ignorant if we would not admit that we have one problem: <u>we cannot rule ourselves</u>!

Regarding all phenomenons of homeopathy, their nonlocal and synchronistic patterns, they may appear to us as the most interesting aspect of science, but I assure you, there are more interesting things than what we can discover between heaven and earth. A life span of just 120 years would never be enough. Imagine what other phenomenons could be discovered when one lives eternally. Astronauts dreams to discover new stars and planets, oneironaut dreams to discover his or her dreamscapes itself and the subconsciousness as even deeper regions. Wherever one's desire to travel ("*naut*" from astronaut is Greek and means "*sailor*"), time, a lot of time, eternal time, gives us all possibilities. So, what is now the real liberty? A lie of being independent from God or the truth about our true nature? You decide!

In this regard, materialists' restraints themselves in every possible way, become slaves of lower frequencies, missing opportunities to learn higher truths and "*mind over matter*" as a natural byproduct of this understanding. Never feed a pearl to a pig, they will not understand nor appreciate. There was a good reason why so many alchemists encoded their observations and insights in a symbolic language. Why care about the ignorant? They will not understand, they don't want to understand. Even the etymological roots of the word "*understand*" will make you "*comprehend*" it's very meaning. It means "*to be in subjection of*" or "*under the rule of*", a "*mutual agreement*". But ignorant people are "*not open to any agreement*" and so they naturally lack knowledge and insight.

Let's return once again to the "*mind over matter*" phenomenon. Mind is higher than matter. We say it's "*frequency*" is higher, because we perceive it like a vibratory nonmaterial stream. And matter is of a lower frequency, because it is low enough to be perceived by our biological organs, eyes, ears and tactical senses. Mind cannot be perceived by the tactical senses or by our eyes, they don't share the same frequency. A higher frequency can affect the lower one, so the mind is able to form, or inform the matter. If the mind is free from illusions which bounds it to lower states of matter, than more it is able to inform and form and exhibit a force over matter. Then it is not ruled by matter, but it rules matter itself.

CHAPTER THIRTEEN

Memory

"You don't need to forgive if you have forgotten,
because it is the same!"

One last phenomenon is the memory of the illness. A patient once came to a homeopath with several complaints, headache and stomach pain and a lot more symptoms, but her headache was her main concern. The doctor visited her, made an accurate anamnesis and the prescribed her a remedy in a high potency, single dose.

After few weeks the doctor met the patient in a shop and asked her how she was doing. She replied that "nothing changed". Ok, that's strange, the doctor thought, because he was so sure that he prescribed the perfect similimum to her, and so he asked a more detailed question: „How is your headache?"
"My headache? Oh, it's gone! I almost forgot that I got this terrible headache!"

The headache was her main concern and the reason why she visited him. Now this doctor is a man of great curiosity and he didn't let her just go away without scrutinize accurately about this phenomenon of *"forgetting her headache"* and what exactly she meant when she said that *"nothing changed"*. In order to not appear like a stalker, he invited her and her husband for dinner together with his wife. At the evening she told him that what didn't change was *"everything else in her life"*, meaning all the little problems and worries, to be honest just a way to say, it was just *"small talk"*. But regarding her headache, she really forgot and it didn't come again in her mind that she got this one big problem. Together with her headache she also forgot her emotional problems, because she harboured a grudge against her sister for decades. With time the headache and stomach problems developed and both, her emotional and physical problems, hindered her to have a more happier life. She really tried to *"let go"* but she was not able to. The similimum, the remedy similar to her inner state, helped her to release this blockage made of condensed energy. Once released this energy is available as an extra energy to the organism. It does not carry anymore the information of the grudge with it and it raise to a higher frequency. Now the memory is like it is forever gone.

In TCM the lung and large intestine meridian has the function of transforming energy from outer source and digest it. A grudge is a condensed part of this information which cannot be elaborated further. It becomes stuck energy and this blockage leads to many other secondary symptoms (stomach pain, headache, obstipation). You can observe a shallow breathing or the breathing is stuck in a person who is unwilling to forgive. Their necks have a lot of tension and their shoulders are very stiff. The contrary can be observed in children, they breathe freely and deeply into their belly and guess why they have so much energy! They do not invest any of their energy in remembering unnecessary griefs or offenses. Well, later when they become adults they have already made a lot of bad decisions and experiences, so this will build up the tension you can observe only in adults. But children should be for us a very good example how to treat each other. They laugh about each other and about themselves. For example, when they fall, instead of crying they laugh. The pain goes away fast with this type of "*reverse breathing*" or at least they don't think any more about it. They continue to play as nothing happened. Imagine that your life could be like that. Someone offenses you, but you let just go and forget the "*transgression*", not why you do not care, but because you know that it will not change anything if you hold it inside you. Letting go means to know instinctively what is of higher and what of lower frequency, what is good to integrate into your system and what is just waste material.

I made my personal experience once with Hydrastis canadensis, a remedy known by certain Native American tribes of North America for cancer treatment. It helps to release a deep condensed energy inside the "Ren Mai" meridian, a energy channel which stores energy and eventually leads the abundance into the biggest storage facility called the "Dantian". I took the remedy in a C200 potency in the evening and the next morning when I woke up I was astonished how deep I could breathe. There was this indescribable sense of "hope", that from now on everything will be fine. And another sensation was inside me, that I finally was able to forget and forgive. Cancer is an illness with the main theme "*I cannot forgive*". They have no energy because they invest all in the persistence of dark memories.

Memory can be inherited from parents or it skip one generation. This happens when the trauma was deep and severe. One generation is not able to elaborate it all, so it is forwarded over to the next generation. It seems that it does not matter who elaborates the memory, when at the least someone would elaborate it for everyone else. Again, there is a nonlocal phenomenon here. And the language of this memory is not an abstract one, but a symbolic, like described in chapter 3.

Bibliography

Gerald Pollack, Ethan Pollack
Fourth Phase of Water:
Beyond Solid, Liquid & Vapor (2013)
978-0962689543

Patricia Le Roux
The Actinides in Homeopathy (2012)
978-3941706644

Jan Scholten
Secret Lanthanides (2015)
978-9074817165

Homoeopathy and the Elements (2016)
978-9074817059

Wonderful Plants (2013)
978-9074817202

Peter Chappell
Emotional Healing with Homeopathy:
Treating the Effects of Trauma (2003)
978-1556434297

Edward C. Whitmont
Psyche and Substance:
Essays on Homeopathy in the Light of Jungian Psychology (1993)
978-1556431067

Louis Klein
Miasms and Nosodes: v. 1: Origins of Disease (2009)
978-3939931683

Rupert Sheldrake
The Science Delusion:
Feeling the Spirit of Enquiry (2012)
978-1444727944
Morphic Resonance:

The Nature of Formative Causation (2009)
978-1594773174

Michael Talbot
The Holographic Universe (1996)
978-0586091715

Robert Becker, Gary Selden
The Body Electric:
Electromagnetism And The Foundation Of Life (1998)
978-0688069711

Dr. B. Sahni
Transmission of Homoeo Drug-Energy from a Distance
(1992)
81-72021-135-2

David Peat
Synchronicity:
The Bridge Between Matter and Mind (1987)
978-0553346763

Richard Milton
Forbidden Science:
Suppressed Research That Could Change Our Lives (1995)
978-1857021882

Charles Seife
Decoding the Universe:
How the New Science of Information Is Explaining Everything in
the Cosmos, From our Brains to Black Holes (2007)
978-0143038399

Dean Radin
The Conscious Universe:
The Scientific Truth of Psychic Phenomena (1997)
978-0062515025

Entangled Minds:
Extrasensory Experiences in a Quantum Reality (2006)
978-1416516774

Amit Goswami
The Self-Aware Universe:
How Consciousness Creates the Material World (1995)
978-0874777987

Massimo Citro
The Basic Code of the Universe:
The Science of the Invisible in Physics, Medicine, and Spirituality
(2011)
978-1594773914

Robert Lanza, Bob Berman
Biocentrism:
How Life and Consciousness are the Keys to Understanding the True
Nature of the Universe (2010)
978-1935251743

Bernardo Kastrup
Why Materialism is Baloney (2014)
978-1782793625

Ami Ronnberg, Kathleen Martin
The Book of Symbols: Reflections on Archetypal Images
(2010)
978-3836514484

George Yule
The Study of Language (2015)
978-1107658172

Bernd Senf
Die Wiederentdeckung des Lebendigen:
Erforschung der Lebensenergie durch Reich, Schauberger,
Lakhovsky u.a. (2003)
978-3930243280

Peter Tompkins
The Secret Life of Plants (1989)
978-0060915872

Ahmed N Currim
The Collected Works of Arthur Hill Grimmer (1996)
978-3929271058

Peter Deadman
A Manual of Acupuncture (2007)
978-0951054659

Damo Mitchell
Heavenly Streams:
Meridian Theory in Nei Gong (2013)
978-1848191167

David Twicken Dom
Eight Extraordinary Channels Qi Jing Ba Mai:
A Handbook for Clinical Practice and Nei Dan Inner Meditation
(2013)
978-1848191488

Stephen LaBerge, Howard Rheingold
Exploring the World of Lucid Dreaming (1991)
978-0345374103

Duncan Laurie
The Secret Art:
A Brief History of Radionic Technology for the Creative Individual
(2009)
978-1933665429

Nick Franks
21st Century Radionics:
New Frontiers in Vibrational Medicine (2012)
978-0957311107

Edward W. Russell
Report On Radionics (1974)
978-0854350025

Alexander Hislop
The Two Babylons (2012)
978-1440070990

Immanuel Velikovsky
Worlds in Collision (2009)
978-1906833114

John C. Eccles
How the Self Controls Its Brain (1994)
978-3642492266

Recommended websites

Homeopathy

- system-sat.de
- homeoint.org
- interhomeopathy.org
- qjure.com
- narayana-verlag.com
- johnbenneth.wordpress.com
- hydrogen2oxygen.net/en
- radionicsnews.wordpress.com

112

Contact

Email: isuret.polos@gmx.net

Manufactured by Amazon.ca
Acheson, AB

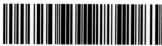